REEDOO

(A beginners guide to practicing the art of Interception)

By

Pastor/Exorcist Sharon L. Flesher

All Contents Copyrighted. Reproduction is Prohibited.

ISBN: 978-0-9844893-1-2

Foreword

REEDOO is simply **extreme** intercession. It is the art of using a visual aid (in this case a tiny replica of a person) to intercede for others. Why did I choose that name to describe it? Because you are redoing what the devils have done and not just pleading/interceding in their behalf but destroying the devil's plans for others.

in·ter·cept *(v. in´tər sept´; n. in´tər sept´), v.t.*
1. to take, seize, or halt (someone or something on the way from one place to another); cut off from an intended destination: *to intercept a messenger.*

How many times do you feel you need a do-over? That is why the first REEDOO experiment by you is going to be 'you'! That's right and you will be amazed at the things that begin to take place as you hold yourself in your own hands and begin to declare the Word of God over your own soul.

If you follow this guide closely and earnestly you will find that you are able to affect the world around you in a new positive way. However, I warn you, do NOT try and make people into what you want them to be according to any selfish desires. If you do that, you will harm your own being and I will explain that in detail within this book.

The art of blessing and cursing is alive in everyone you know and we all practice it to some degree. You are doing it right now as you read this by your response to the information by either condoning or condemning me and what I say. Most don't realize what they are doing and many of us think little about what we say or do concerning others in our private lives and contemplations. We tend to believe that our *words and thoughts are not heard by anyone but us and we ignorantly believe that they just fall innocently to the ground....they don't. Every thought produces a frequency and we will speak more of what that means as we go along.*

Please do not skip to the instructions on how to make the doll(tiny person) without reading the book. You need to understand the mechanics behind the spirit world to not harm anyone or yourself. I call this method a step beyond intercession and named it **interception** *because you are intercepting the devils vibrations and casting them out whilst removing the damages done and restoring healthy vibrations to the body and sending positive energy to assist those who are being attacked by unclean spirits. Everyone emits energy as we all have spirits.*

If you would like to leave a testimony after practicing REEDOO, please visit us at <u>breadandwineministries.org</u>. You may leave a testimony on our forum, ask questions, or you can reach us through the contact page.

Thank you and God Bless,

Sharon

REEDOO

(A Beginner's Guide to Practicing the Art of Interception)

Contents

How it Came to be..2

What is REEDOO?...6

Negative Energy (Demons)..15

Positive Energy (The Holy Spirit)...20

Understanding Communion (Unifying With God's Spirit)...............................32

Understanding Fasting...38

Understanding Spirit..41

The Meditation..54

What You Need...59

The Blessing and Deliverance Process..64

Preparing Items for Use...80

Group Sessions..88

The Patterns..100

The Journal...102

How it Came to Be

Having studied and practiced deliverance techniques for well over 25 years, with my first deliverance miracle at the age of 13, I realized the need for helping others from a distance. Also, our internet ministry thus far has grown by leaps and bounds and I ashamedly admit that I reach countries I've never even heard of before. We reach people behind iron curtains and people who are too timid to talk to others about their problems or their faith and this has my heart struggling for ways to help them. How can you go to all of them, pray for them, lay hands on them, cast out disembodied spirits, and heal them? They e-mail me and I cannot go to them...I thought....or.......can I?

So after crying out to God on how to deal with this, this revelation struck me like lightening. "Thank you Jesus!", was the exact words from my mouth as I wrote the details of the process down that I saw in my spirit. Like manna from heaven, these words will change the lives of all who partake of it and are able to receive it! (This information will also be taught in even greater detail in my seminars so if you ever have a chance to attend one you might heartily consider it.) I've learned that when you grow in Christ everyday and His mind is constantly being imparted you will never lack for understanding and all that you need is provided and you find yourself overflowing with blessings and wisdom. Christ's mind is infinite and one can never reach or encapsulate his mind or truths in one book or even thousands. This world cannot hold Him and certainly it cannot contain all of what He is capable of doing through our own lives. Think of the infinite possibilities! Much of mankind lives in a box type mentality and by that I mean that we confine ourselves to small statements of faith when in fact God is Faith itself and is infinite.

Therefore, man must come out of his box. He must leave his gender, his culture, religions, and his preset notions behind in order to grow in Truth. The heart must come from the right place and then nothing is impossible to man as long as He is aligned with God.

What this book contains is just one broad aspect of how your spirit works and how to help aid those around you. You can of course pray for anyone without a little doll or object to represent a person but just as Paul's handkerchiefs and the hem of Jesus' garment changed lives, so will your with your tool of faith! By faith it will be created and by faith it will be used as a visual aid to manifest healing and deliverance to those who need it most. It will also give you a place and point of contact to administer healing. Before you judge me as to whether or not this is of God, please read the book and see the revelation for yourself. Healing may well come to those whom you bless and your life will be blessed in the process as you hold your own self in an objective position of prayer, speaking words of faith and truth over your own soul.

Take your time reading this book and the purer your heart becomes, the stronger your positive energy, and more successful you will be at this. I suggest doing Communion (the proper way as described in this book) before you attempt to do group deliverance and it would be ideal if each member attended a group training session to familiarize themselves with the process so it will work smoothly and seamlessly like an army going into battle. Again, take your time and move from true love and you will see things you never before could have imagined!

Many of us have loved ones who are dying spiritually as well as physically. It isn't the death of the flesh that is as traumatic to the individual as the movement to the lower realm upon death and leaving your flesh behind. This shift in vibrations is painful to the spirit let alone the realization that your body has really died and yet you are not dead but not in heaven either! Imagine your body failing along with your religion...... both are painful beyond words to a soul.

You can combat the dark energy that is pulling your loved ones into darkness and contend for them. Don't let the ones you care about on earth just slip away into oblivion without so much as a struggle! Take a stance and be ambitious in what you know is right. Now is the time to act upon your convictions while the people in your life are still in their bodies.

This revelation came to me as people began dying around me and as I watched some of my family and friends being pulled away by demonic forces. In these end times the love of many is growing cold. We must form a strong alliance of truth and true resistance to negative forces in order to function well as the body of Christ and to not become those who practice Churchianity instead of true Christianity.

Like I said, I was crying out to God one day about the enemy and this revelation lit across my mind with visionary strength. I already understood the power and application of intercession prayers, and then on the negative side, the power of the voodoo dolls and how disembodied spirits are sent and used to inflict torment on others. I knew this even though I never practiced voodoo. I also was fully aware of who/what unclean spirits are and then it all came together.

So take your time digesting the information in this book. This is a spiritual book so when you feel your mind is full just put it down for awhile and come back to it when you feel hungry again. These revelations come to you through hours of soul searching, blood, sweat, and tears and are more precious to me than my own life because they are from God's mind to me.

It is wise when searching for Truth that you meditate and learn to give your attention to God. This process is also on my website at **www.breadandwineministries.org**. *Many cannot give their attention to God because they are literally in a hypnotic state by devils. This is due to reacting wrongly to situations and wrongly to what is going on within themselves and can only be cured by true repentance which will never happen if one cannot view a situation clearly. Meditation will open that door for you if you really want the truth.*

You see, the further you pull from that which is not real, the closer you are to that which is Real (God) and we are the children of Is-Real. We must not seek what is not of Truth. To seek such is to seek the face of demons. God is Truth. All that we do must be from what we understand not from what others tell us we should do. We are to be Spirit led not unclean spirit led.

Therefore, ask the Father to open up your heart to understand this and it will simply make your heart sing for joy as you enter into the kingdom of heaven within you!

What is REEDOO?

REEDOO is an art in itself; like prayer and worship. It is 'way' beyond what is commonly perceived as intercessory prayer by most religions and people. The fundamental concept is that you are going to visualize the person you are about to intercede for and you have a 'point of contact'. You will begin to send them positive energy as well as perform deliverances (casting out devils) from a distance with extreme success and you will change the lives of those you intercept. How this happens will be explained as we go along in the book.

"Why the doll?", you may ask. I will tell you. The doll gives you a point of contact. You will be able to use anointing oil, lay hands on it, sprinkle holy water, and hold it while praying in tongues, etc. Plus, you can visualize that person easily by placing a photo of them on the face of the doll and adding pieces of their DNA or articles that their essence has entered on to the doll! Your mind won't wander away or be as tempted to stray away and it will be as if they came in person and you are helping them.

Wait! Before you scream, "Yippie!" and grab a doll and run to your prayer closet, let me cover some deliverance techniques that will knock the socks off of you! You will be sending evil spirits away like a pro and understanding what is happening. It is also highly important to grasp the difference between blessing and cursing. Often what we have been taught as positive thoughts and blessings are not blessings at all but confessions of non-truths made over in sympathetic disguises.

Saying things like, "I will win the lottery," may sound like a positive thing to say but is it? If it is said from a spirit of greed do you think it will *turn out well? Probably not! So we need our thinking to line up with the Truth in order to speak it and change lives in a positive way. Where your heart is at must be understood before you grab a doll and start pumping out words without understanding. Muttering things you've heard others say can be devastating. You can really harm people by sending them negative energy in prayers. In order for God's energy to become manifest in another person's life the words must be from God Himself. We must speak in accordance to God's Truth or we will be sending others negative energy and destroying them even more!*

In Voodoo you send someone strong negative energy/spirits. You do this by focusing on a negative thought and emotion like anger. This draws strong evil spirits to you. Hate, anger, and loathing are very strong evil emotions. Then, the person who is cursing someone will push a pin in a doll where they want that negative energy to go and release it by emotionally letting go of that anger as much as possible. We don't want to practice voodoo in the name of REEDOO and that will be one of the focuses in this book is really defining the difference between blessing someone or cursing them and helping you find the right place to come from. Otherwise you would be better off to not practice REEDOO at all because if you do it from the wrong place you will eventually die from it because you are drawing death into yourself before you send it onward and then it returns to you again! It is one of God's spiritual laws.

We ignorantly curse people all the time and are presently dying from it in ignorance but this process will speed up our rate of deterioration. When we think and speak evil of someone we often don't realize that we are sending evil spirits directly at and into others. What is worse is that we do this in our prayers and think that God is just like us and 'on our side'. We pray things that are beyond horrible. I've heard of people praying for others to die, for spouses to do what they want or to obey them, and for every lust under the sun! People stand up and curse each other in the name of God and walk away proud and even entire churches have been known to gather in one accord and curse! It's like watching a bunch of drunks with loaded guns! Often we don't even know how to stop the 'shooting' as the anger is deeper than our understanding. So we ignorantly and sometimes knowingly destroy other people in our state of stupor and wantonness.

*Okay, enough of that.....let's talk about energy. You realize that there is a good and a bad energy. You can feel alive or drained. You meet someone and you feel your energy pulled away from you yet cannot explain what just happened and so you avoid them like the plague. Sometimes, certain people make you feel alive and you visit them because they always make you smile and you tend to come away feeling almost fuzzy inside. You can't explain it but you like being around some people and you don't like being around others. You may notice that on a more rare occasion there are certain people who can **completely** drain you! You dread seeing them coming and after they leave you feel an immediate need to 'restore' yourself seeking things like hot beverages, baths, and solace. This is evidence of energy coming and going between people or sometimes just 'going'. Notice that it has either a positive or a negative affect on you. Interesting, isn't it?*

Your energy can be depleted or increased. This is what we see going on. What does this and why? Well, my dear reader, you are spirit. Spirit is energy and energy is always either depleting or increasing. It is ever moving like the wind. We are vibrational creatures in a vibrational world and moving 24/7.

"Vibrations?" you ask, "how did we get on that subject?"

Science has proven that every thought has a frequency and all matter is vibrating. There is nothing that is not vibrating and all your senses send their information to your brain through vibrations. Unclean spirits operate on low frequency or vibrations and everything you see is not solid. It is actually over 99 percent empty space!

Therefore you are either vibrating closer or further from where you were designed to vibrate at. This perfect frequency or vibration is the vibration of God's own spirit and is what I call HF or High or Heavenly Frequencies. Ghosts vibrate really low. You can buy meters to detect ghosts. Like I said, everything you see around you is not solid. It is vibrating particles that are made of more small particles and the essence of them is Spirit.

The scripture says, "God is all and in all". And so it is true that all things were made by Him. Not only this, all things are Him! He is all things and as no thing that is corrupt is God, one day soon all that you see will be gone. The earth is set to be renewed as God will make a new heaven and a new earth and all low frequency vibrations will be done away with and disposed of (eternal hell).

What we are going to do is speak to things that are not as though they already were. This is what faith is. We are going to move from God's word and move mountains effortlessly by changing the vibrations just as He does. After all, it is Him in us that is doing the work if we come from His Spirit.

16 For by him were all things created, that are in heaven, and that are in earth, visible and invisible, whether they be thrones, or dominions, or principalities, or powers: all things were created by him, and for him: 17 And he is before all things, and by him all things consist.

Col 1:16-17 (KJV)

There are two laws or principals of God we are going to look at. One is the fact that matter affects matter. Imagine matter as one perimeter of vibrations and then spirit is faster, slightly offset to it. All matter can affect matter. Rain falling on dry dirt can make mud, for instance.

Another law we see is that spirit overrides, affects, and changes the vibrations of matter. All that you see, is and was created by Spirit. The Father's Spirit knows no time or distance as He is everywhere at once. Therefore, you don't have to shout for Him to hear you. It was Spirit that hovered over the waters that had already been created by Spirit and it was Spirit that brought our world into being and it was our spirit pulling away from the Creator that lowered it into corruption. What feels solid to us does so because we vibrate according and in tune to it. For instance, unclean spirits can feel each other but can only feel this world through us because they do not have a body anymore to sense its vibrations. Which is why they long and seek out people to inhabit.

God is a Spirit (John 4:24). He is not an old man sitting on a chair somewhere in the clouds wondering what is going on below Him. He is everywhere at once and knows all things because He is all things. That being said I want you to realize that we are made in His image. This means that you are not in your body, your body is in you. Your spirit is creating the 'new' you everyday. Every time you move from a thought that isn't of God, you pull dark energy into your being and your vibrations begin to slow down or change. Every time you move upon God's thoughts your vibrations increase and draw nearer the way they were meant to function, bringing you health. If you were to perfectly align and not move from a negative thought or emotion you would simply vanish by vibrating according to the All Spirit God and be like Enoch or simply ascend like Elijah did. Of course you would have to do so according to God's will as that would be the only way to move in perfect unity with Him and stay on HF thoughts. Jesus had perfect unity but was sent on a mission. When the mission was complete he was transfigured and he left. "My life is in me," he said.

Seeing as we are all here right now (me writing and you reading) we need to realize that we have a ways to go before we do not move from even one Low Frequency type thought. Therefore, there is no need to esteem ones self above another. Instead, it causes us to understand how important it is to seek the mind of Christ and to have that Mind imparted to us instead of the thoughts and ways of those spirits who are headed to eternal doom.

*If you practice REEDOO from a negative energy you will not be practicing REEDOO anymore but Voodoo and that will eventually cause you to get sick so please pay attention to where your heart is at. Gradually you will recognize in yourself what spirit you are coming from. Remember this one rule '***where you come from determines where you are going***'. If you come from a Low Frequency thought or emotion God will not be behind what you say or do. The angels will not uphold the words of demons or any LF thought. Who will come and aid you in your efforts? Those who sent you the thought in the first place! That only leads to more sickness, more sorrow, and more separation from the life giving force we seek.*

Therefore, if you want to bless someone you must move from God's mind and emotions in order to accomplish it and you must be able to recognize and resist the thoughts that are not His. This happens over time and you need to give yourself room for mistakes as you will most likely make your share of them along the way. You must speak the Truth with your understanding as it is imparted to you. The more you do it the easier it becomes. This isn't as hard as it sounds and I will give you some ideas and things you can safely say that are powerful. But I want to cover first some of the wrong places that you can come from and give you a heads up on what is transpiring when you speak or pray for others.

We cannot be the Light. This is a very humbling thing to discover inwardly. We like to think of ourselves as a deep well of great power and mystery but the truth is that we transmit what we hear and we are not the source of anything. That would make us God and we are not. Therefore, we cannot be our own understanding. We can't just go decide to forgive anyone and make their sins disappear, then wield a big sword and cure the world right after our cup of mojo of course! Pride gets us into so much trouble. We like to imagine that the world revolves around us and that we are amazing, worthy, astounding, powerful, and worthy of adoration and we are not. God is all....that leaves little room for anyone or anything else to boast. Until we get a little humble and see the role we play in creation we will continue to promote demonic thought in the earth, and even do it in God's name — to our shame.

*Jesus said in John 8:28, "**.... I do nothing of myself; but as my Father hath taught me, I speak these things**". This is how you must be. Taught of the Father and speaking of the Father. Once you begin to come from that place, your words will not fall to the ground because they have 'meaning' to your heart/spirit and your spirit will be moving in unison with the all powerful God and you will be an extension of Him in the earth. The angels will uphold all that you say because you've said it from faith and by understanding what it meant. When we don't know something, we must say, "I don't know" and wait for God to show us and quit trying to become our own answers, cease rote memorization, intellectualism, and give up pride food.*

So in every instance we are either hearing and moving from His voice or demonic voices. Do you see the importance of coming from the right place in your heart and speaking the with words of Truth from your lips? You are made in the image of God and just as God creates from His Spirit, you create from yours. If you want to kill someone you can just be angry at them and if they don't have angelic protection your anger could eventually make them sick and kill them. Especially if they are not protected of God. It will eventuallykill you too because there is another spiritual law that you have enacted upon yourself, unbeknownst to you. Namely........

Cast thy bread upon the waters: for thou shalt find it after many days.   **Eccl 11:1 (KJV)**

Here we see that what you are sending out is coming back to you. Therefore every LF thought or unclean spirit that you send out comes back to you. Most likely with more energy than it left as the person you dislike usually dislikes you too. This is what is often called a 'cord' by some people. It is an interlinking of spirits between two or more people that can only be broken by repentance and true forgiveness of at least one of the two who are tied together. When an interlinking is present if you are paying attention you will notice that you and the person you dislike seem to know a lot about each other and things that you shouldn't be able to normally know. Often you will hear each others thoughts and view each other, finish each others sentences, etc. This is very common as you both are connected in the spirit realm by one or more spirits who are tattling and stirring the pot of evil in you both. Only by non-participation in LF thought betwixt the two parties can this cord be truly severed. You can command it severed in Jesus name, but it will only be temporary and restored to function the next day. Similar sins make a cord strong and keep it bound between two people. Spirits travel on back and forth on that same frequency that both people are using and even just one lonely little spirit is able to argue against itself to cause trouble and fights. They are very crafty and cunning and not hindered by space and time.

How do you travel if you are a spirit? By thought of course. Have you ever thought of someone and then had them call you? We all have! When you think of someone you trigger their spirit. Just try this. Look at the back of anyone's head and begin to shout at them mentally. "Hey! Look at me!" Make sure they are not focused on anything really intensely. A perfect time is when someone is drifting off to sleep or sort of sitting quietly. Shout it over and over at the back of their head without them seeing you and do it in your mind and watch them spin to face you! Astounding how it works so easily! How many times have you 'felt' someone watching you to turn and find you were right?!

To sum it up. All that you see comes from Spirit and is vibrational. Spirit changes matter, even evil spirits do this....remember its still sin (wrong thinking) unto death. Your spirit has functions. These functions/ways create your world as you know it now. Spirit is all....and all is Spirit.

The point I'm trying to make here is that our world is not as it is often perceived and in the spirit world if you visualize someone and think of them, you are connecting and connected and influencing that other spirit one way or the other. This is one reason the REEDOO process really works if done correctly. You are making spirit connection and changing their world for the better!.......Wow......Let's continue.

Negative Energy (Demons)

Before we get into making the doll and the aspects of the deliverance and prayer I want to talk about your real heart. This is the very center of your being, not the organ that pumps blood to your body. That one only represents the real one. Why do you want to do REEDOO?

If your reasons aren't right it will come out all wrong for you. I don't want to see this happen. You can't do REEDOO to 'make' someone agree with you or to make your world a better place for your own comfort. It must be from real love in your heart or not done at all, otherwise you are practicing black majick. Seeking to control other people for your own benefit is the heart of all witchcraft and dark arts.

Here are some underlying thoughts and emotions that will turn REEDOO into Voodoo:

- *anger*

<u>Thoughts like</u>: *I'll show him, who does he think he is, how dare she say that, we will see about that, he will do what I say, she will obey me, I'll make him forgive me, etc. Any form of punishment on an individual is wrong. We are not to judge or condemn....only to send positive information to the heart and spirit. We don't hate anyone we hate sin (wrong thinking). There is no need to hate because God's Laws are in place dealing with every person under the sun. He is fully aware of all His creation and no one or no thing will get away with any evil thing...this includes you!...fear God..... Resentment must go along with spite, revenge, and hate!*

- *selfish reasons for prayer or praying for self advantage*

<u>Thoughts like</u>: *Once this person gives their life to God they will really love me, this person is so mean to me...I have to change them to like me more, etc. (Self gain is the main thing to watch for. Stop trying to take care of yourself and give your situation to God and it won't haunt you anymore.)*

- *greed*

<u>Thoughts like</u>: *God wants me to be happy, I will pray over myself to get rich! I will confess that I own six cars, three houses and all the chocolate in the world! I am amazing, beautiful, and worthy of adoration, etc!*

- **Lust**

<u>Thoughts like</u>: *This person will marry me. I am commanding her to love me and give her life to me in Jesus name. (all love spells and thoughts are FORBIDDEN! Nothing says, "I'm a creep" like trying to control and manipulate another soul for sex through a tiny little doll on an alter!)*

- *Envy*

<u>Thoughts Like</u>: *She will suffer for what she did to me. He will be sorry. God will punish you. Your sin will not go unpunished. (Basically any statement made from bitter envy or jealousy). Thoughts that say.....Look how spiritual I am praying for your pathetic little soul. "I have you in my powers muh ha ha!!!!!" These are FORBIDDEN!!!!!*

- *Arrogance*

<u>Thoughts Like</u>: *You're so little and I'm so big. I have you in my hands now!*

I will control your future! You have to do what I say now. I'm right and I'm going to prove it to you now., etc. or any kind of thoughts that promote the ego in you or others is strictly prohibited.

- ***Spite***

<u>*Thoughts Like:*</u> *"Oh, yeah?!.... this will teach you a lesson! Mess with the bull and you get the horns! I'm taking you to God and you'll be sorry. I never get mad...I get even! "…...(Any kind of revenge will lead you to disaster). Real love doesn't want to harm anyone and always does what is best for the other person.*

- ***Self Pity***

<u>*Thoughts Like:*</u> *"Even if you don't love me, I love you. One day you will see how much I really love you. If only I could rip my heart out and hand it to you, then you would see how wonderful I really am." Any place where you come from a 'poor little me' thought, self pity is flourishing and self pity is a LF emotion. If God is taking care of you, should you be complaining? I don't think so! There's never a good reason to feel 'sorrow' for ones self. It insults God and is demeaning to others.*

All these examples are Low Frequency thoughts and emotions. If you move from them these LF waves will return to you and when they do they bring dark or negative energy into your spirit which creates sicknesses on your body and unclean spirits or energy waves make you vibrate too slow causing your body to break down and God's life force energy is cut off from you.

Everything that is wrong with us has a perfect cause and a perfect cure. That cure of course is God Himself. The cause is sin or wrong thinking that we act on which is separation from God. In order to begin to change our energy and others we must begin to move from HF thoughts and ways and project those ways into others. (HF stands for High Frequency or Heavenly Frequencies).

Instead of sending LF to people we must send HF. This is why real love is so powerful. I'm not talking about 'like' and 'hate'. That is the two headed dragon of death! I'm talking about doing what is best for someone without regard for yourself. You know that kind of Love because He came and showed it to you. He left everything for you, died, and does what is good for you even now as you read this and for what? What does He need from you? He is everything. He did it because it was what you needed. This is how we are to be towards others. At the very least we ought to love our fellow man as much as we love ourselves. We would never knowingly kill ourselves with LF. Therefore, now that we have the wisdom to know the dangers of LF, lets begin to hunt it down in us with a passion in our souls so we may be the pure in heart who see the Truth!

"How can we do that?", I hear you asking. We can do it by examining our hearts every day, living completely to what we've been shown, and trusting the blood of Jesus to cover the rest by grace as promised. I want you to listen to my audio file on communion as I don't want you to partake of Jesus' blood unworthily. It is on the website. Also it will be explained briefly in this book.

*When beginning the practice of REEDOO, I want you to first make a doll of yourself. I want you to make a journal of how you feel about you and what you are praying over **yourself** first. This will help guide your heart in the way that you will help others. You may find that once the doll is made and you have turned it into you that you don't like the doll or that you are* *uncomfortable around it or even hostile towards it. Write everything you feel down. You may also notice that you now have become aware of yourself in a special way, an almost unnerving way. The reason you are uncomfortable is that your mind has become awakened to observe yourself from a distance and this is actually good for you but a bit scary for those who like to hide. Please mediate in between your prayer sessions. These will help you and the Father will guide you into the truth and God Himself will speak to you there as well as throughout your day as you come more fully into the light within you.*

*Some people will feel that the doll is looking at them or is all of sudden.....evil. Your recognition of spirit entities as powerful can easily be projected into the doll. Believing in your own false power only encourages your imagination toward the darkness. We are not pulling any spirit into the doll but using the doll as a means of contact with the living— not the dead. The doll is **not** to be worshiped or feared, okay? It is like a 3-D photograph and nothing more. Please don't make the doll out to be more than it is. It is a tool that we are using for positive energy just like you use holy water or oil! You aren't afraid of water are you or your anointing oil? Then you have no reason to be a afraid of the doll. We aren't calling evil spirits into the doll in this book although we will be battling them through it in some measure. We will respect the doll as we respect all of God's creation but we will not worship it and one doll may also be used for many people which I will explain all that in greater detail as we go along.*

Now that we have covered dark energy somewhat I want to speak to you about positive energy and give you some examples to draw from. Later on I will give you a list of things you can say so that you have somewhere to start when you begin to practice REEDOO.

Positive Energy (Holy Spirit)

If you want to send positive energy you have to move from God's thoughts and emotions. What is God thinking anyway? What is He feeling?

God isn't a human being. He isn't made in our image. We are born with wrong thinking and are corrupt. Even our bodies must be redone one day so we can dwell with Him. He is perfect. He has 'never' sinned. Not even once! Awesome! No wonder He is worthy to be worshiped! It is impossible for Him to practice wrong thinking....... Therefore, if you wish to move from His Spirit you must be as united with Him as much as possible and especially during REEDOO for your words to have any punch or positive effectiveness. The goal? His words coming through you. Think of it this way. Satanist break all ten commandments in order to endowed with demonic power. We are going to keep all the things that God has shown us in our hearts and in doing so, God will uphold us as we are in unity with Him and moving from our understanding.

Positive Energy then is really God's Spirit moving through you. This is why it is imperative to spend time meditating because it will unite your heart to His gradually over time in a way that cannot be easily undermined or destroyed by devils. Watching (observing) and praying (wishing) for the Truth is the only way to not enter temptation (that which is not true). Put your faith in His power, not yourself. You are a vessel. See it. Fill up, pour out.

Begin to seek God on what to say and do during REEDOO. Ask Him to show you the pains of the person you are praying for, the thoughts that you need to rebuke, and the spirits that you are up against. Ask Him to reveal

His nature and His mind to you concerning the person you are about to pray for. Seek scriptural references from Him concerning yourself and others. Wait silently till you hear a verse and then turn to it and ask for understanding. Fill up....pour out. Forget about the ego man. He's fake. Focus on the Father.

Also, begin to observe what is going on in your own life from an arms length instead of getting caught up in it and losing yourself in problems and situations. Watch yourself make mistakes, feel the grossness of it and don't try to fix it but stay in that helpless state and wait for Him to come and rescue you—He will and it will be a rescue indeed! Notice that you don't have solutions and in doing so you won't possess the problems and the problems won't possess you. Wait on the Lord....look to the Lord....follow the Lord. Give up making decisions. It's a foolish conquest. Only move when you see it is right and let paths unfold.

*When you are in an aware state you can linger in those moments where a temptation comes front and center and you will find that He is there to sustain you in those moments. You will feel the pull of darkness and see the tricks of the enemy and be able to **not** participate because of the emotional distance you have from them. It is when we are caught up in the scene of things that we are not able to separate from them and we become part of the made up story that spirits feed us and we live in their dark confused minds. We move from pride (their lies of who we are) which causes us to try and fix things, create things, and rule things. Tossed by every whim and scheme of the dark minds around us we live in frustration and stay fixated to thoughts and ways that are all LF. Worry is a sign that you have taken up a problem as your own and are in your pride to fix it. Don't try to create an answer. Are you God? Then what in heck are you doing!?! Wait for the answer to* *come to you. God will simply impart it when you need it. God didn't give you your problems....you took them upon yourself! Give them back and quit playing god and you will have peace. Fill up....pour out.*

God is willing to show anyone the Truth. Pride is what keeps us in the dark. It is what stops us from seeing that we are doing wrong and repenting. Is pride worth it? Is it really worth living for a lie if the lie and you both perish? Yes, it hurts to know the truth about the things you do and have done, but the pain of seeing that first burst of light is well worth the vision you receive after you step into the light! Oftentimes it feels like you are dying, but it isn't you that's dying but the dark spirits that have told you that you were them! The real you is growing more and more alive every day as long as you are seeking and moving upon what God reveals, one day you will awaken in His likeness and truly be a brother to Jesus! Glorious!...... and praise the Lord!

In REEDOO, to do it correctly and without harming yourself, you need to understand what positive energy is. If you make a mistake and speak something over the doll that was not correct, simply recant and begin again. Ask God to forgive you and take it back. God is merciful and will forgive you if you are sincerely sorry.

Here are some examples of positive things you could say as you pray or extend your spiritual energy to another. These are assuming that the person(s) you are praying for are saved. I will not delve into deliverance techniques until later on. Basically you will notice that I am prophesying over the doll. I am speaking things that are not as though they were because in Christ we are a new creature created unto good works and God's Spirit is our Spirit and is the real Self or identity that we are to identify with. Remember, you are standing on the truth, becoming at one with the Truth.

Truth that is revealed to your inner man will be the most effective words spoken.

Positive Statements:

- *You are a new creature in Christ Jesus. All things are passed away and all things have become new.*
- *God has not given you the spirit of fear, but of power, love and a sound mound*
- *Your spirit is not weak*
- *Your spirit is not sick*
- *Your spirit is not fearful*
- *You are repentant of your sins*
- *You obey God in all that you do*
- *You love the Truth*
- *You want the Truth*
- *You serve the Truth*
- *You do not identify with dark spirits*
- *You will serve God all your life*
- *Your words are His words*
- *Your ways are His ways*
- *Your mind is His mind*
- *You are one with Him*
- *You have the Spirit of Power*

- *You have the Spirit of Love*
- *You have the Spirit of Peace and a sound mind*
- *God is in you and you are at one with Him*
- *All thoughts and ways that are not of God are not of you*
- *All your needs are met*
- *No devil can destroy you*
- *No sickness can overcome you*
- *You are covered by the blood of Jesus*
- *You are not afraid of anything*
- *You are protected by the angels*
- *Everything you do is upheld by the angels*
- *Cursed is everyone who comes against you to destroy you*
- *Blessed is everyone who blesses you*
- *You are not blemished*
- *You are not diseased*
- *You are not alone*
- *You are the righteousness of God in Jesus Christ*
- *You are the body of Christ*
- *You love the Light*
- *You do not love sin*
- *You do not seek devil's minds*
- *You serve the Truth with all your heart*

- *God is in you right now*
- *You are not evil*
- *You are humble*
- *You are kind*
- *You are unselfish*
- *You do not boast*
- *You do not seek to please your flesh*
- *You have given your life to the Truth*
- *The old man has died and you are alive in Christ and a new creature*
- *Jesus is your King*
- *You bow the knee to the Truth*
- *Love lives in and through you*
- *God loves and lives in you right now*

Base what you say upon the truth revealed to your heart. Say it by faith. Calling things that are not yet as though they were. When you hear tongues interpreted, tongues that are prayed in behalf of one's own soul, they sound like those confessions mentioned above. They are confessions of truth. What is occurring is that as your mouth speaks out the truth, even though your conscious mind does not usually comprehend it, your vibrations are changing because of it. This begins to bring life to your spirit as your vibrations increase so does your anointing or presence of God. It is like a small yellowed plant reaching desperately for the sun. The photosynthesis does not occur all at once but over several days — often years for us!

As God begins to reveal to your heart who you really are in Him it will help you to pray the truth over someone else. I definitely suggest that you do NOT pray for people you have not yet forgiven or to pray only from good feelings with carefully preordained phrases. You must become aware of the emotions behind the words. Begin to learn this art over your own doll first and then branch out to others and do it from the right place in your heart.

If you move from anger or hurt and hope to change someone so they will be what you want them to be so you can get what you want out of them, this is dark energy moving. Secretly you are hoping that they will love you or obey you so you can use them. This will only end up cursing you both. Selfish ideals and emotions are not easy to avoid if you don't have anything else to move from and odds are your statements in REEDOO will have a margin of error. But be consistent in seeking God's guidance and that margin will decrease! This is wondrous and one needs to start with a doll of ones own self to learn it correctly.

Please realize that all prayer spoken from evil intent is a form of casting spells. When someone who is angry with you for disagreeing with them cries out, "I'll pray for you" in arrogant overtones. What they have actually done is threaten you. They are saying, "I will curse you" but in an overtly nice religious way.

If you are not angry with them, their curse won't stick to you and you need not fear any angry person, a devil, or evil's ways. The demonic spirits curses(pigeons) they send to you will have no place to roost and they will return home to the sender! It will bounce off of you and simply return to its sender if you don't hate them or resent them for being a misinformed soul. People who practice voodoo are also aware of this and are instructed to 'release' their anger or the spirits will return to them harming them instead and if they accidentally curse a real person of God, they usually die whilst

God's child remains unharmed. Why? They would have to destroy God to get to you because you are at one with Him. Also, if you get angry and try to harm a true child of God you are toast! Most people die within a couple of years when they put a heavy hand against God's anointed.

As I said before, I don't want you to fear spirits. They have been around you all your life and if they could instantly kill you, I assure they would have already. I see demons when I do exorcisms sometimes and God protects me because I do not do it for my own gain but to help others and so He is there in the process. I also see angels and I'm telling you that you are easily protected and have no reason to fear unless you are seeking demonic ways and thoughts. Only by your own faith and belief of the devils thoughts and ways, only these empower them in your life. That is why they try to make people fear them. They slam doors or shake curtains and make noises. If you really fear them they will attack you but they are only able to do it because your fear (which is faith in them) and it feeds them. Generally speaking, it is you who empowers them. They must have your energy, as it is stronger than theirs at this point in creation, to do any sort of evil deed to you. You must turn off their access to your energy by turning your attention to the Father instead of to them. All you have to do is begin to confess the Truth and move from it and God will overpower anything they try to do to you. You can also 'project' that positive energy upon them and they will run like heck! Meditation will extend your spiritual energy and you can feel the power exiting your body and environments as they are pushed back. By allowing the Holy Spirit full access to your heart, mind, and soul, you can and will destroy negativism in your life and others. Generally speaking, one must never engage the demonic spirit in your mind or in conversation in an inquisitive or fearful way. One can simply either rebuke them and ignore what they are trying to teach you and focus upon hearing God's voice instead. This will begin to annihilate the effects they are having on your life and close the door they are using to 'get in'. Resist the devil and he will flee.

Unclean spirits often move when it is dark. The reason evil spirits tend to move in the dark is because the dark has less resistance to their frequency. Three or four 0'clock (in your time zone) in the morning is the easiest time for them to move around. Also on full moons the magnetic pull helps them. There are also times when planetary alignment is in their favor as far as their vibrations and energy go. They are LF and have to work around God's creation to move and do things.

There is no reason to fear demons as long as you are seeking God. God is not afraid and He is more than able to protect you from harm. Put your mind on Him and the fear will fade into the dust from whence it came and all the little spooks will fade away too.

Now that we've covered some positive thoughts I want to reiterate that the world's version of 'positive thinking' is not necessarily positive. Saying over and over, "I will win the lottery" so you can have a lot of stuff and let devils live through you vicariously is not of God, okay? All negative thoughts are thoughts that are not God's and all positive thoughts are ONLY those thoughts that originate in and of God.

Think of the possibilities. Not only can you minister to your own soul but you can carry around a sick person's doll and pray in tongues; sending them direct energy. You can anoint them with oil where they are ill at and command healing in Jesus name. You are not limited to a 'one time visit' at a hospital or interrupted from helping by horrible weather or continental divide. Your budget won't stop you from ministering and neither will distance. You can pray every day for your husband or your wife, your children, the pastor, the president, or the neighbor. You can lay hands on the sick and be there as there is no time or distance in God and the more positive energy you emit, the more you receive! So pray, pray, pray! When your brain gets tired, just kick into autopilot and pray in tongues.

Realize that our minds bring things and situations into our lives. **You become your thoughts.** *If your thoughts are corrupt or if a corrupt spirit triggers your thoughts and you do not resist, then you will succumb to that corrupt thought. What if you could intercept those LF signals that are attacking your brother or sister? How would it change their lives? Is this what Jesus meant when he said he 'kept' his disciples?*

Let me ask you this, are we one body? Do we have a right, and even an obligation to keep our brothers and our sisters? Does the devil have the right to make us sick seeing we are in Christ?" No! Devils have no right or authority over us anymore if we are in Christ and living unto the Truth in our hearts. The only reason evil spirits are able to destroy us is because we are ignorant and allow it or are really not in Christ in the first place (our hearts are not given to the Truth). In which case repentance needs to take place.

God expects you to put on your armor and fight. He expects you to go in and possess the land(spiritual places) He gave you. You are not to sit idly by and watch people die and say, "gee, I guess I"m next...too bad for me". No, God expects you to move as He moves. To bind up and help the brokenhearted and set the captives free and to break 'every' yoke! You can start with yourself. He told us to cast out demons, heal the sick, and raise the dead. Those are 'action' words.

Although I am an exorcist and face demons, God has so far blessed me with an ability to simply not fear demons of any size or kind. It isn't that I'm super brave or anything or really mighty or strong of myself. Actually it is just the opposite. I know that I'm nothing. I have no degrees to brag about, no famous friends or recognition by the world or churches standards, and I don't really want them either. I tried that shoe and it doesn't fit. I don't belong there. Those matters to great for me and I prefer the simple life. I know that it is only God that keeps me and that it is only God that is wondrous so I find that I cannot care who likes me or what they think of me and still be able to help. How can I help someone if I am trying to get something for me in the process?

I understand that I cannot do anything of myself....... and this is my strength. Although this is a growing revelation, I have come to understand that what I once viewed as my enemy, that which attacked my ego, was really my friend and that situations I use to avoid that could and do often end embarrassing or demoralizing are most often those that are best for my soul.

When people shake their heads at you or feel really sorry for you in a degrading way, treat you badly, ignore you to hurt you, or esteem themselves above you, it is actually really good for you if you take that to the Lord in prayer and do not return evil for evil.

Do you resist evil to 'prove' that you are good? Don't do it! Let everything be exactly what it is without struggling, let your life flow naturally like the brook. Only move when the Holy Spirit shows you that you must and then move from Him in you and you will know the power of God in your life. As long as it is all about you, you will become all that you will know, and this leads to spiritual disaster and you will become your own religion and trapped within an endless loop of thoughts.

Our strength comes when we abandon the hope of another power to save, deliver, or preserve. Therefore, deliverance ministry is for everyone and really all real ministries are deliverance ministries because salvation is deliverance from evil. Again, every person who follows God is into deliverance and by that I mean they are actively involved in leading people away from evil to that which is good. The Truth sets us free and so it is with exorcisms but it is a much more 'in your face' approach. There are just times when a demon isn't quietly working behind the scenes but boldly killing someone and cursing and ruining someone's life and you must take action. The really malevolent ones know no shame and need a firm hand.

Although I am fully aware of how to confront demonic spirits and how to force them to comply, we will not be taking the doll thing in that direction. Instead we will simply do remote commands which are really effective and have proven to bring healing and deliverance. One of the strongest things you can do is command someones body part to obey you and it will. Like, "I command the heart to beat normally." Confrontational exorcisms, where a person is full manifest, will not be covered in this book.

After I cover communion I will explain what things we need to construct the doll and then how to do a deliverance and effectively use the doll. Communion is a powerful and important tool because the purer your heart the more powerful your words will be. And remember, visualization is what you are after. You must picture it in your mind. You must see the person in the place of the doll when you are ministering.

Just as illnesses must first form in your mind before they enter your body, so does healing. It is by our faith that we are healed and it is by faith that mountains move. If you wish to move a mountain in the life of someone else you must see it first. That is why this method is so effective because it links you to the one you are ministering to in a nonthreatening objective manner and you can minister whenever your heart is led to do it.

Understanding Communion

(Unifying With God's Spirit)

The word 'communion' means to interchange or to share thoughts and emotions. It is intimate communication. You can only keep real communion if you understand the principles behind it, otherwise it is just another mindless ritual that leads you to a purple tongue and a bad snack. The audio file on my website on communion will help you but it will be briefly explained here as well as it is an integral part of ministering and doing REEDOO as it helps unify you with the Father/Truth.

Jesus took their supper which they were about to partake of together and picked up their bread and said, "Take it and eat it, it is my body which is broken for you." He broke one loaf and shared it amongst them all. He then took the wine and said, "This is my blood which is spilled for you. Drink ye all of it."

The bread represents the embodiment of Truth/Jesus. He did not sin. Which meant that he did not move from even one wrong thought. What you are doing by taking the bread and putting it in your mouth is signifying that you want the truth in your mouth. You are partaking of the truth. If you do this unworthily it means that you are lying to yourself and others and not really wanting the truth but wanting to look holy by taking the truth into your life but not moving on it. This is how to get sick. True communion is done by examining your heart in the Light of God's presence and then 'repenting' or turning from your error to the correct thought.

For we *being* many are one bread, *and* one body: for we are all partakers of that one bread.   1 Cor 10:17 (KJV)

The blood that courses through your veins when you give your heart to the Truth is now the same element that gave life to Christ. It is the Spirit of God that you are partaking of. You are to partake of 'all of it'. Not just the parts of Truth that your ego, the false you, wants to see. Look at this comparison below.

Ye cannot drink the cup of the Lord, and the cup of devils: ye cannot be partakers of the Lord's table, and of the table of devils.   1 Cor 10:21 (KJV)

Paul is saying that you cannot partake of a devil's spirit and God's Spirit and be a well person! Why? Can you follow lies and truth simultaneously? No! No more than you can go right and left at the same time. Therefore either one or the other has your allegiance in any given situation and one or the other sits at the root of all you do and at the root of your very health or illness. If you seek the truth but really love lies, you will get sick and die for you are partaking of Him unworthily.

What you are aiming at here by taking communion is singleness of heart. For only the pure in heart will see God—the Truth. Therefore, what you desire is to weed out anything in you that is not of Him; any deception, any wrong thought, motive, idea, or emotion. These are all the enemies of Christ in you and we don't want to be found as a cohort with devils, loving them, listening happily to their lies, and snuggling up to them like bosom buddies. Are we not the bride of Truth....betrothed to Him for all eternity? We must seek to unite with the Spirit of Truth.

Your central reason for doing Communion must come from a revelation and understanding that all the ways that are not of God are a waste of time, life, and energy. Every belief that is based on wrong thinking will perish one day. If your life is based upon these wrong thoughts, emotions, and ways your soul will also perish with those LF thoughts.

In others and those that you pray for this is also the case and the main reason people are sick. They are moving from dark energy and their spirits are too weak to bring health to their bodies and their lights are going out! Step in and begin to increase the amount of positive energy in their life. You can intercept the negative energy and project God's thoughts, emotions, and energy to them and it must be a 'continual' process throughout your day with your mind. We are to pray without ceasing.

29 For he that eateth and drinketh unworthily, eateth and drinketh damnation to himself, not discerning the Lord's body.

Here we see that if we don't discern the truth in ourselves yet or identify with it in our understanding we are partaking of the Truth 'unworthily'. This causes us to suffer. When we see the truth but then promptly denying it because it hurts our pride or we don't think it will give us some such thing we secretly desire, we deny His voice and choose the 'other' voice. This immediately begins to bring damnation or dark energy into us.

30 For this cause many are weak and sickly among you, and many sleep.

31 For if we would judge ourselves, we should not be judged. 32 But when we are judged, we are chastened of the Lord, that we should not be condemned with the world.
1 Cor 11:29-32 (KJV)

Most illnesses come from us drawing dark energy into our spirits. God knew that we would not be able to come into perfect understanding all at once and so He gave us grace and continues to do so as long as we stay on our quest to find and know the Truth in our beings.

If you would be able to properly see the Truth in you and follow Him, you would not be condemned because you would repent and turn to obey the Truth in your heart. This would cause your spirit to emit HF as God's Energy/Spirit would flow from your spirit. To enter HF's you have to repent or turn from the LF's. Refusing to see the Truth will result in physical and spiritual disaster!

Only those who are led by God's Spirit are His sons. The fact that you must be led means you have not arrived yet. So realize that all people everywhere have some level of LF thoughts, emotions, and ways moving in their lives. This is the same as saying that unclean spirits/ghosts are accessing every single person you know, giving them thoughts, moving their emotions, and causing sickness in some level or degree in 'every single person on earth!'.

For every spirit that is successfully shut down through Truth, freedom and healing comes to that individual in the area of your spiritual energy that they were draining. You can help the body of Christ the same as you help yourself. You have legal right to do so! Are we not all One in Him? Am I not a part of you and you a part of me? We are indeed our brother's keepers!

Now, having the understanding imparted to you of the real meaning and keeping of Communion what I want you to do is do it physically to reinforce what your heart now knows.

Go get some bread (any kind) and wine or juice. Set the bread before you on a platter and ask God to examine your heart. Sit quietly and listen. Focus on the light behind your eyelids and set your intent upon the Father. Ask Him and beseech Him to reveal to your heart where your faults and wrong thoughts are at. It may take you a while and your bread may become stale but you must seek the Father's face to see Him, right?

Then, once you see and repent, take the wine or juice and drink it. Know that you are being led by the Spirit of God. This is your life now. You are not following the old you anymore but the new you which is Him in you. The person who sought to know himself as god, loving lies, pride, and ego was not the real you at all but an imposter trying to live through you. You are a new creature in Christ, born of the Truth and are at one with Him! You have just partook of the very life blood of Christ....the Truth. Then take the bread and eat it. This represents that as He laid down His life, His body was broken for you, so you are to forsake your own flesh. You are now taking part of His thoughts and ways instead of the devils thoughts and ways. Do you see why doing this in a lying way would lead to sickness?

You can also practice Communion everyday before you eat your meals and use the food on the table to represent the principals behind Communion. This is what the meditation does three times a day! It sits you in the presence of God and allows you to come into the Light. I will give you a brief understanding of the meditation here but please visit my website at ***www.breadandwineministries.org*** *for the full version.*

The meditation isn't hard but for it to be effective in repentance you must come from the right place in your heart when you do it. You must want the Truth more than anything in the world and want it for the right reasons. If you want to get deeper into deception it is a powerful tool much like daydreaming where you can make things that are not true as out to be real to you in your imagination. This is what the bible calls evil imaginations.

But they hearkened not, nor inclined their ear, but walked in the counsels and in the imagination of their evil heart, and went backward, and not forward.   Jer 7:23-24 (KJV)

This will be you if you do the meditation from emotions that are not pure. For instance, if you desire to become really spiritual and powerful and amazing or if you seek to stand out amongst the crowd by unifying with the Almighty and seeing yourself as a 'cut above' the others as His 'special' person. What you are doing in a round about way is seeking glory again! The ego is at it again! These kinds of sins will peel away from you one layer at a time and exposed by the Father as you are able to bear the truth. The sincere heart will find the Truth and as long as you honestly want the Truth you have nothing to fear and no harm will come to you from meditating. All things will end up working out for your good and you may well fall a thousand times but your Father, who Father's all who love Truth, will come and pick you up.

We cannot help but move from the wrong information that we have and each wrong belief/understanding must be replaced with correct understanding. Keep seeking, asking, and knocking on that door of Truth and you will find.

Understanding Fasting

Fasting has long been known as a method to purify a soul. At about the third day you can feel yourself shrinking on the inside and pulling away from the living. It is really a humbling process because you get to feel your frailty and it is an generally an 'ego' busting process. I like to fast often but for short durations. I feel that each person must move in accordance to their own heart and faith. I do know of people that are so hard-hearted that fasting only serves to establish their already inflated ego! They actually fast to prove how amazing they are and how they are more spiritual than others. This makes fasting pointless and you will damage yourself in the process.

Fasting is a lot more than not eating or drinking anything. I do usually drink on my fasts but some people I know don't eat or drink. Legally I suppose I should mention that you should consult your doctor if you decide to fast.

Fasting is really the act of your spirit humbling itself as it comes to realize that it is nothing. Something about feeling all your greatness threatened and starting to perish seems to bring things into perspective. Never fast to prove a point, change someone else out of pride, or do it to feel great, powerful, amazing, or spiritual in an arrogant way. These are all LF thoughts and emotions and your fast will hurt your health if you come from an LF thought. I wish doctors knew this and could ask people why they wanted to fast and only allow or approve of those who have pure motives. To fast for wrong reasons will hurt you and so you've been warned and I can guarantee that if you do it for any other motive than a right one that it will come back to bite you in the end!

Now, another important aspect to fasting is that you need to do it in the secret confines of your heart. This is also evidence of a correct heart stance. Don't go around moping, complaining, looking longingly at food, or seek sympathy from others for all the great suffering you are enduring for such a noble cause. Why? Because you will lose your reward. "What reward?", I hear you asking. Why your revelation of course! The answer to why you are fasting! If you stop eating to seek the counsel of another person or to gain some sort of spiritual notoriety you have defeated the purpose of fasting, received your reward in earthly terms, and your heavenly revelation will not come to you. Do you realize that you have fasted unto man and received your reward from him instead of God? This isn't going to strengthen your spirit but weaken it. It will just encourage you to become really religious and make you believe that you are so dedicated and amazing and worthy of worship that people must recognize you. It's just an ego trip when done in the flesh and of demons and by demons.

Your reasons behind fasting must be the same as the reasons you keep the real Communion. In this case however you are not only seeking to destroy evil in your heart but are crying out to God in a special way. You are forsaking the world in you and outside of you! As you refuse what it feeds you and look only to the Father with pure intent to draw near Him, He will bless you with revelations and tons and tons of hugs and kisses!

It isn't easy to fast for three days or more. It gets really hard when you are hungry, dizzy, or weak to not seek the sympathy of man or the eyes of those around you. It takes practice to not get angry or upset when you are tried and yet you are weak and tired and then required to do things such as cook a full course meal for your family on an empty stomach and to do so without feeling any sorrow for yourself in the process. If your heart isn't set clearly on the reason you are fasting, you will get angry and sin in your fast. Real fasting is like the triathlon that you train for as you work out between the Communion and the REEDOO. It is the event that seems to pull it all together, bringing strength into your walk with the Father as your soul becomes more humble.

Successful fasting is really humbling and cleansing to the soul. I have actually grown more fond of my fasting days than the eating days because of the amount of revelations and 'hugs' from heaven! Only the humble and the contrite dwell with God and this is where you want to be. This is where you MUST be if you want to send Positive Energy to someone else you must come from God in you. This is why fasting in the flesh is so damaging. People do it to brag. "I fasted for 40 days", one person bragged and then I found out later that they dumped all their food into a blender and sucked it through a straw and called it fasting so they could brag. Think of the pride it took to come up with that delusional scheme! Shame on them!

Please read my 'How to Fast' pdf on my website to gain further insight on the subject of fasting. Like all things in life you get out of it what you honestly put into it. Put self into it and self comes right out! Polished and shinny and ever so grotesquely alive. Put truth into it and Truth will come out of it and out of you and your inner Light will light the world and set it on fire for the glory of God. Praise God!

Understanding Spirit

What is Spirit? We touched on this earlier but will go a bit deeper now.....It is everything as it is God. Spirit creates matter and moves matter. Eventually all LF will be removed from the land (Zech. 13:2). We will live forever in HF's but for now we are living in corrupt vibrations. Salvation only comes from pulling away from the LF vibrations. This is what is commonly known as 'going to the Light'. As there is no corruption in God and He is everything, all that you see and know that is corrupt will one day be 'gone'. It is like a passing dream, a fading flower, and dust in the wind.

Who are we and what is our spirit like? I can only give you that which I have been shown thus far. God is a Spirit (John 4:24). We are created in His image. Is His image corrupt flesh? Are you your body? Yes and no...and let me explain. Your body has come about by LF vibrations. Our world is vibrating lower than it use to when it was first made. Adam and Eve were 'removed' from the garden upon sinning. This lowered their vibrations and they entered a world of corrupt people. Cities were already there as Cain was afraid he would be killed. These were not nice people in this world that Adam and Eve had entered. Whether it was fear or sorrow that kept them near the spiritual portal of Eden, I do not know.

However, this never changed the fact that our spirits operate as God does. So what does His Spirit look like? We see it in Revelations as God speaks to the 'whole' spirit of man.

And out of the throne proceeded lightnings and thunderings

and voices: and there were seven lamps of fire burning before the throne, which <u>are the seven Spirits of God</u>.

Rev 4:5 (KJV)

God has Seven aspects to His Spirit. You do too. These can even be felt. Please read 'How to Be a Spiritual Christian' for more in depth details. Basically, every energy point that you have is described as the churches in the book of Revelations. I prove it in my book 'How to Be a Spiritual Christian' and when these energy points get sick your light or energy begins to dwindle.

Tiredness or lethargy for no apparent reason can mean demonic entry into your energy points. They drain you and deplete your vital life energy because they corrupt your vibrations and inhibit HF from moving. Like a radio dial that isn't quite on the station you fade in and out and are not receiving energy clearly. It isn't that devils have negative energy or a power apart from God but that they align you to incorrect vibrations which lowers your vibrations and depletes you. This is why it is sin unto death....or wrong thinking until the real you goes to sleep! Their corrupt minds which are not awake to the Truth put your mind to sleep with theirs. Do you realize that you are becoming either at one with the Truth or at one with what is not true on a gradual basis as we speak? You are making progressive steps in either direction..... waking up to see the Light or going to sleep with those who are in the night.

These seven aspects or 'churches' that you have can be represented in the ceremony, named, and spoken over and prophesied to if you desire to do so. As your understanding grows so will your prayers and effectiveness. Just start simple and then let it unfold as you grasp revelations. I will describe the Churches or Energy points briefly and then you can bless them accordingly and rebuke spirits in accordance to them. It is important to realize that your body is simply reflecting spirit activity that has come and gone in your life. Demonic spirits that accessed you have much to do with everything from your appearance to your currant state. We cannot help that we are accessed which is why the bible says we are 'born in sin'. We are born into LF's. These negative vibrations twist, bend, and corrupt everything from your basic DNA elements to your mind/spirit. We are inundated with wrong information and programming in both areas from the time we are conceived! Only by God's Spirit can we be realigned unto pure vibrations. We can't align ourselves as we aren't the source of Power/Energy.

Salvation is of the Lord/Truth. By believing into Jesus you can be saved. His blood/truth covers your sins. He died in your place, for you, so you don't have to. But in order to receive salvation you must repent of your sins and live unto the Truth in your heart. Grace covers what you don't know. But God fully expects you to obey Him in the revelations He has imparted and will put all who don't obey far, far away from Him. You must be obedient to what He personally has shown you, not what others tell you that He says, but only that which He Himself by His Spirit in you has revealed to your heart. This is how you can be perfect as He is perfect and fulfill the commandments of the Father in you. When you live like that you enter the kingdom of heaven within you and you will know you have arrived for the overwhelming joy and peace in your heart! Oh my gosh! Sometimes it is a physical force that takes my breath away and there will be no guessing as to whether or not you are saved. You experience that salvation now! You enter heaven now! If you aren't living there now, you won't go there when you die so knock, seek, and ask and strive to enter those straight gates of Truth.

Lets take a look at the seven aspects that your spirit has. This is also why there are seven aspects to the armor of God because you must protect your spirit in order to be well and safe in Him. Your spirit overlays your body and spirits can feel each other and are solid to each other. You don't own things in the unclean spirit world but you do fight, maim, torment, and inflict pain on others. It is a very 'dog eat dog' world. Things are different in that you don't have a physical body that has limitations. Just imagine how our world would change if no one was tied down to a body? Would anyone be safe in their homes? Would money stay in the bank? Would you be able to shower in peace? Probably not! No wonder spirits wander and seek rest and enter people!

In my book 'How To Be a Spiritual Christian' I cover in detail what God said to each of these energy points. Here however, I will cover the meaning of each name as He gave them. The candlestick He will remove is the energy that your spirit is emitting. It will 'go out' if you do not repent and do as He has commanded in each of these admonitions. For reference see Rev. chapters 1 thru 3.

Ephsus:

The 1st Energy point that you will notice is at the base of your spine and is called 'Ephesus'. The word 'Ephesus' means 'first desirable'. This represents the first time you desired to really see the Truth. If this desire is based upon a corrupt reason, this energy point will get sick or be sick. Sicknesses associated with this area often are people who have 'left their first understanding of truth' and suffer emotionally in the following areas. They frequently have panic attacks, suffer from extreme fear, have a self preservation mind set, are extremely insecure, and often are very resentful of *others.*

Health wise their lymph system, skeletal system (teeth and bones), prostate gland, sacral plexus, bladder and elimination system, and the nose (because it is associated with survival) also may suffer and they are weak physically in those areas.

This energy point is along the spine at the base of the spine. You can anoint the gown in that area, pray over that energy point and claim it for Jesus. Command any negative energy to leave in Jesus name. Make sure all commands are in the name of Jesus....this represents your understanding that all lies bow to the Truth. Remember, not all illnesses are from sin. Some illnesses occur for other reasons. Don't take liberty and judge others but observe, pray, and intercede as the Father leads and do it only to bless others and because what you are doing is best for someone else.

Smyrna:

*Smyrna means 'bitter affliction'. When this is not functioning properly it means that you were not willing to suffer for the Truth that you had received in your life. Basically you loved the fake you more that the real You and you are identifying with devils in you instead of God's Spirit **after** receiving the truth.*

Character traits that are noticeable when this energy point is misaligned are a mouth that is out of alignment. Instead of professing the truth to people you sympathize, complain, boast, brag, slander, and mock etc. You knew better but weren't willing to suffer in your flesh for what you knew and gave into the momentary gratification that comes with sin. When you receive demonic thoughts as your own, the only way to separate is to 'see' that you are wrong in your understanding and move upon what you see. Often people aren't willing to suffer for what is right for fear of what it will cost them either physically or emotionally. They often forgo the truth for momentary pleasure that sin provides. Unwilling to lose friends, positions, and family, they cave to demonic thoughts and ways.

Sicknesses in a person's body generally reflects what is happening in their spirit. For instance, if you are refusing spiritually to reproduce the words of God and the revelations He has imparted, what happens to your body is that you can no longer reproduce. Reproductive organs get shut down. Sexual problems, such as perversion or even failure to be able to perform when needed are also signs that your 2cd energy point is not functioning properly. Liver failure can also occur, kidneys, lower abdomen, and the lumbar plexus are often affected by heavy demonic entry at this point. So if your mouth is out of whack in a way that it won't hold on to what it knows is right, it means that this energy point is being severely depleted by LF. If you want healing you need to begin to suffer in the flesh. That means that you must begin to obey His voice in you and close your lips in humility and contrition and suffer from partaking of that moment of pleasure that comes from disobeying God/what you knew was right. It takes revelations to do that or it will just be another act of pride!

See why meditation is so important? You can't go out and buy that revelation at your local mall nor can you study and 'achieve' it. You can only find the Truth by seeking Him and He imparts Himself to you. **It is not in your control to perfect yourself.** *You can only seek and God will reveal Himself to you as you are able to bear the Truth in your heart. If you cannot receive the truth for pride's sake, then you will only be religious like the pharisees and not holy like Jesus. Your knowing will always be simply* *head knowledge and your faith will be dead and all your wondrous works will count for 'squat'!*

Pergamum:

Pergumum means 'earthly heights'. When this one is out of whack you are usually in big spiritual and physical trouble. This is the place where you can actually feel demonic activity. It occurs in your solar plexus and associated nerves. Quivering sensations, that 'sick to the stomach' feeling, and nausea feelings come directly from this place. Also the 'gut' feeling that seems to mystify most people occur here as well, proving that we can have the Holy Spirit guide us from there as well as demonic spirits. Do you know why? The reason there is so much activity here is that you have a stomach brain and spirits are energy and use our brains. Babies function fine without a cerebral. Their bodies develop first and the brain last. People without a cerebral have been known to stay alive proving that the stomach brain is fully capable of controlling our bodies functions. The stomach brain is also known to effect our emotions considerably and some scientist believe that it may be responsible for all our emotions which is another reason to begin to separate from our emotions in order to observe them. We must be sure we are moving from correct emotions so as not to entertain the wrong spirit.

We actually have three brains according to our scientist. We have a small heart brain, a stomach brain, and a cerebral. Unclean spirits can use these just as we do because they know how to. They were once with a body and so there is no learning curve for them. When I do exorcisms, demons generally come up from the solar plexus. It seems to be sort of nesting ground for them.

In order for this energy point to function well you must 'rise' in frequency above the earth's frequency which is why it is called Pergamum by the Father.

The character traits of those who are getting really dark in this aspect of their spirit are people who are generally motivated by anger. These tend to enjoy hurting others for no reason, manifest dark blinding rage, have frequent temper tantrums and fits (which are really manifestations), and are often obese. They cannot contain their belly/lusts. The illnesses they generally have are muscle issues, stomach, digestion, pancreas, liver, gallbladder, metabolism, and the nervous system. Pancreatic cancer, nerve disorders, gastric problems, renal, testicular, and spleen because dark energy is depleting the life force that these body parts need in that area.

To pray effectively for that person, you must begin to anoint that energy point and lay hands on the stomach area. You can also command the demons out in Jesus name and I will get into that more later. Next we have.....

Thyatira:

This energy point is near your heart and all the energy points are in alignment along your spine which is as you know many nerves which act like a highway for energy. Thyatira means continual sacrifice. This is what must happen to have a heathy 4th energy point/heart. The heart must let go of what is not real that it once loved. It makes a continual sacrifice of its 'self' to see the Truth. That is what a 'healthy' heart is doing. A heart that is not doing this will soon suffer heart stroke or disease, irregular heart beats, etc. Some kidney functions can also be affected because of how the kidney and heart function in unity. Hole in the heart, irregular heart beat, and high blood pressure are all signs that one's heart is not completely given to seeking the Truth. Heart disease is considered the number one killer in America and its source is linked to stress. Stress is one's heart not trusting *the Father but trusting its fake ego self, Just as our spiritual hearts are failing, our physical ones simply follow suit.*

Character traits that are prevalent when this energy point is being bombarded with dark energy are a double tongue, fearful words, worrying, stress, and things like drinking, smoking, and such things are signs of a troubled heart. We often use these to escape our convictions/hearts and try to drown out our Conscience by turning up the volume on the television set and the world. Music, constant reminiscing, problems, and planning the future are always ways we try and escape the present moment that pains our awareness of guilt. Becoming extremely intellectual is another way to escape the truth. It is our way of becoming our own light. We believe that we just aren't smart enough to overcome a problem and so we set out to be the light instead of receiving the Light.

Sardis:

Sardis is located at the base of the throat and means 'prince of joy'. When in alignment it would be confessing the Truth and glorifying God. Signs of its malfunctioning or darkening are mouth and throat cancers. It can also cause weight gain just like the Pergumum. Other illnesses may include the thyroid gland and all neck and throat areas. A person who spews out demonic nonsense on a fervent basis is setting themselves up for these things. Teeth issues may also be connected and many of these things are still in the process of being discovered. Basically your mouth is more than out of alignment, it is down right ugly and out of control! You can see how some symptoms and issues overlap. Our spirits and souls are complex and intricate.

Lets take a quick overview of the five aspects I have covered and I will show you a healthy spirit man being formed:

- ***Ephesus**>first desirable> Your first desire to see the Truth birthed a new creation. Your heart cry to Jesus to save you from your sin.*
- ***Smyrna**>bitter affliction> Persecution for seeing the truth came to you....you held your ground and suffered for what you knew was right.*
- ***Pergamum**>earthly heights>Because you did not move from dark spirits and you did suffer instead of give in, you rose above their frequencies and ways.*
- ***Thyatira**>continual sacrifice> As long as you continually make that sacrifice you will continue to grow in Him.*
- ***Sardis**>prince of joy> This is you entering into God's approval of you which brings joy to your soul, no guilt, and you feel His smile.*

Are you seeing the road map to heaven now? You must first desire the truth, then not run away from what you see. You suffer at first because your ego is pained by what it sees much as ones eyes are pained by the light when coming out of a dark room. Then, when you don't run but confess and hold on to what you have been shown and make that sacrifice of your ego you enter into the kingdom of heaven. What next? What happens next is all but amazing!

Philadelphia:

Philadelphia means 'brotherly love'. Did you know that you cannot really obey the Lord's commands to love until you've already went through the first five phases? Brotherly love, real love, is never selfish. It always does what is best for the other person and does not consider itself as part of the equation. When a person is in full denial of Truth and refuses to repent, lives only in the past or the future, and rejects God completely they suffer dementia, Alzheimer, panic attacks, and mental disorders. They also practice their wrong emotions...hate, lust, jealousy, selfishness, and self preservation.

If you find a person who once knew a lot of truth and then they 'changed their mind' and went with their ego instead you will see that they will begin to experience these symptoms. You will see it for yourself if you only observe. Don't seek to gain some kind of elevation in your observation. That will be you suffering from your own dementia!

Laodicea:

Laodicea means 'people's opinion or people judged'. If this spiritual energy point fails you will be demonically possessed and not just oppressed but fully taken over and probably not even aware that you have become them. You may also suffer brain diseases, tumors, and clots, etc. Any malfunction of the cerebral. They can also suffer neuro diseases and nerve disorders.

Signs of a complete malfunctioning Laodicea is everything from complete insanity to brain disorders and usually becomes full obedience to demonic spirits if you don't die from the brain illnesses first! A sick and dying Laodicea will begin as a person who is highly intellectual in a egotistical way. They usually secretly believe they are amazing and gods and are just awaiting an opportunity to prove it to the world and get the homage they *crave. What happens is that they have not judged within themselves correctly. They saw the truth but did not repent and so all their efforts are based on 'getting away' with the evil they love and they think they can 'work' the system to their advantage. Most who do this are highly intellectual people or people who are born already damaged by those kinds of spirits.*

A well Laodicea will begin to receive direct messages from heaven! Because you've entered heaven through true recognition of truth, repented, held on, and waged the battle of faith, held your tongue, and loved as you should have....then entered the joy of the Lord, then.......your Father speaks to you. WOW! Can you say WOW!?! This is truly the kingdom of heaven within!

Do you see why it is so important now to sit in God's presence from the beginning? To feel His guiding hand moving you through those steps and strengthening you, feeding you, molding you, and guiding you? Praying with your understanding, living from what He shows you, being truly spiritual, not boring, dead, and just religious?

In REEDOO, what you will do is anoint each of these areas on the body and pray over them. You will command dark entities to leave, ask angels to assist and they will hear you as you speak the thoughts of the Father towards them. You will prophesy over each of these energy points. You will do it as you come into an understanding of what you must do and then it will be natural and life changing for those you intercede for. Also, something very important must be said here. Seek God's wisdom 'before' you do any REEDOO on someone else. Your heart must align with God's concerning the individual you are about to pray for. If God has given someone over to a reprobate mind you must not interfere. You must always put 'unity' with the Father first and foremost.

I ask God to tell me where to stand concerning others and then He gives me a scripture or a word and I go from there. Seek the Lord and ask Him to help you know what to do. Then follow your heart with what He gives you and God will overlook the errors of any sincere heart. He loves us all very much and seeks all who worship Him.

The Meditation

Examine me, O LORD, and prove me; try my reins and my heart. For thy lovingkindness is before mine eyes: and I have walked in thy truth. I have not sat with vain persons, neither will I go in with dissemblers. I have hated the congregation of evil doers; and will not sit with the wicked.
Psalms 26:2-5 (KJV)

Our hearts must come from a place of longing for the Truth. Do you realize that without God's mind to move from you only have one other source of information? Do you really want to live from lost minds? There is no right place, wrong place, and then.... your place. You are either living and moving from one source or the other in all that you do. There are low frequency thoughts and high(heavenly) frequencies. There is only good and evil, right and wrong, God's thoughts and thoughts that aren't His.

As there is One God there is also only One Truth. Our perception has little to do with whether something is true or not. If you wish to walk with Jesus who is the Truth, can you associate and have unity with lies? Can you 'twist' the Truth to please demonic spirits and pretend right along with them that you are smart, amazing, and worthy of worship and still be a follower of Truth? Satan fell in love with himself and what did it get him? Is God a respecter of persons? Folks, there is 'nothing' apart from God and if we don't see this in our hearts we will go to be with all lie lovers in life as well as in death. Having made my case, I proceed.

My book 'How to Be a Spiritual Christian' covers meditation in detail if you would like a more in-depth look at it and there are free mediation audios on my website. Here is the sitting position I like the best:

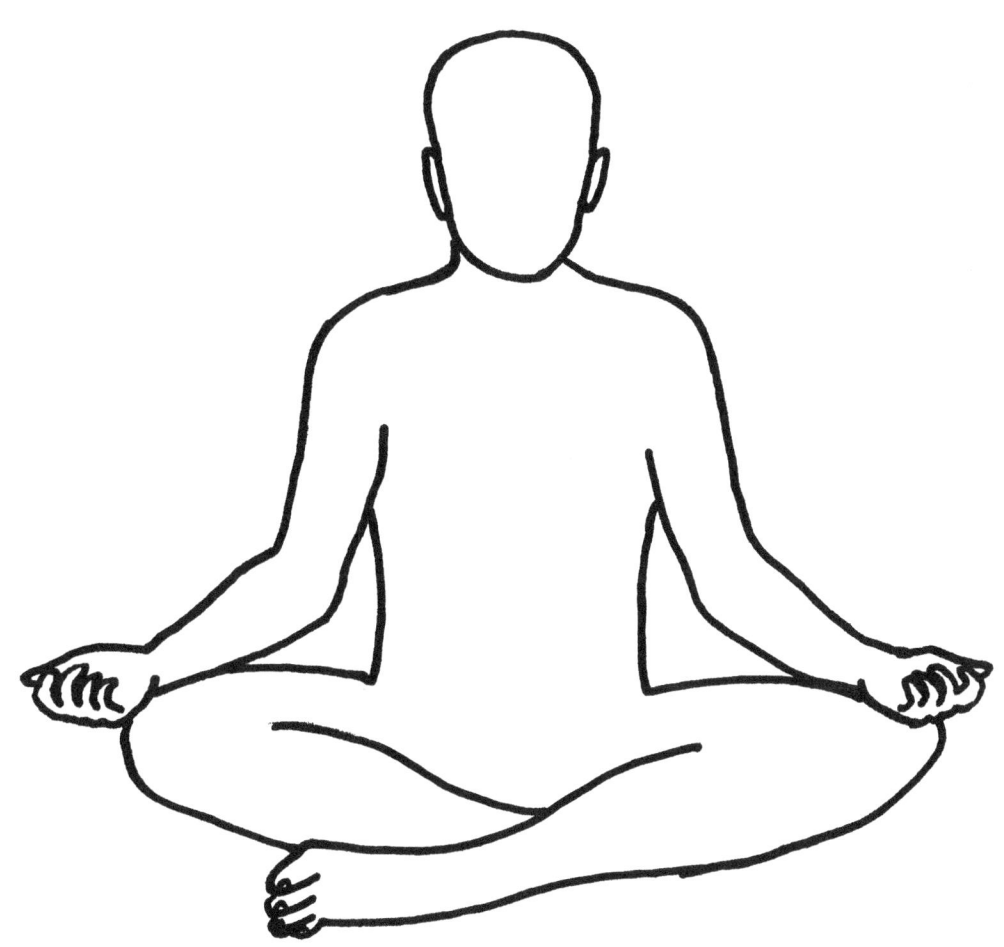

Again, I like the sitting position in the drawing on the previous page. I turn my palms up and relax my fingers so I can feel them tingle. Then I take a deep breath and exhale with my eyes closed. I also love to meditate while lying flat on my back in bed. One must be careful to not fall asleep however and I seem to experience more revelations whilst in the sitting position.

Now, while your eyes are closed, look out into space as if you could see out of your brain through the middle of your forehead. Careful, don't strain your eyes. Notice that it isn't dark! This is the most amazing thing. Just look at the light that you see and pull the light towards you.

Imagine that it is coming in through your forehead and see it in your minds eye trickling down through your neck and on down into your fingers. Feel your fingers tingling. If they don't tingle, just notice your fingers each individually in turn. First on one hand and then the other. Wiggle them slightly if you must. Do this until you are distracted by a thought. Perhaps something that is upsetting to you has pulled you into 'its' thought.

Notice the thought as if it were a commercial or even some other persons thought. View it from the aware position that you now have and pull away from it back to your fingers. Return to the light by looking at it through the middle of your forehead and pull it into you again. Keep doing that over and over until you can control your own mind. This allows you to think objectively.

In most mediation the goal is to blank your mind or shut it down with meaningless chants and dribble. We don't want to do this as it will give demonic spirits more freedom to travel and cause mischief. What we want to do is bring you into the awareness of what they are trying to do and doing within and around you. We want to become aware, awake mentally and stay in the moment where God is at so we can hear Him.

What are the thoughts that are theirs? What emotions are they impressing upon you? You will never know until you become objective to your own thoughts and emotions. Once you break their bonds they will leave and take their dark, energy depleting spirits with them and your healing will begin to occur naturally. So begin to learn how to watch them and they will not be able to trick you into becoming them. As your heart begins wishing for the correct thoughts and ways you will have truly kept the Lord's admonition to watch and pray and you won't enter into their tempting little thoughts anymore if you are awake spiritually.

I suggest three sessions a day but the one in the morning is the most important although I confess I enjoy the one at night the most as I often view things like my own aura/spiritual energy and such. But when you are done meditating, stand up and stretch. The way I like to stretch is to reach up with both hands and then lower them slowly in an outward motion while putting pressure on your arms. If you pay attention as you lower your arms you can feel all your energy points as your arms lower to your side.

You can also do this mediation lying down or sitting in a chair. The reason I like the position I illustrated in the book is because it seems to allow more sensitivity to spirit movement and I am able to stay more alert. If your knees can't take that position try elevating your buttocks with some books or pillows and it will take considerable pressure off of your knee joints. I also highly recommend Roy Masters Be Still and Know meditation. It is excellent for beginner meditation and gets you off to a fast start.

Once you gain the ability to be objective through meditation you can begin to hold thoughts at will and observe them without getting pulled into them. You will begin to 'notice' things like why you did something or why someone else did something. This will allow God to help you through resentment issues and such and help you accept and see the truth in your own life. At first and for awhile you may feel as if you've gotten more ugly. This is because you are becoming aware of who you really have become by moving on wrong thoughts. We cannot change without this vital step and it is because of this step that most stay in the dark. They honestly cannot admit they are wrong or have followed a wrong spirit. Some are too proud to even admit that an unclean spirit can access them. How can they get free?

Again, I suggest doing the meditation two to three times a day. Sometimes you will feel the need to stop and then begin again. Just follow your heart and don't be afraid. Every meditation will be different. I think this fact is one of the most intriguing aspects of the meditation. Sometimes there is relatively nothing going on and sometimes you will see the colors of your own aura and once I had an unclean spirit leave with an electrical charge. You never know. So don't expect any certain thing, just begin the meditation and move forwards in whatever experience of lack of it that God has in store for you.

The heart of the meditation that makes it work is the desire to know the truth no matter what it is going to cost your pride, your body, or your life. This includes being willing to face and see your faults and all the wrong thinking that is alive and moving in your mind and soul! All these are the enemies ground in you! If allowed to grow or develop like a mold spore they will rot you inside out! Be serious in your efforts to meditate.

4 Stand in awe, and sin not: commune with your own heart upon your bed, and be still. Selah.   **Psalms 4:4 (KJV)**

What You Need

Now that we've covered positive and negative energy and how to gain the most positive energy we can through meditation and continual repentance we will begin to gather our items and explain how to use them in the following pages.

What do you need to practice REEDOO?

- *a doll*
- *a fabric cross*
- *a crucifix*
- *anointing oil*
- *container for holy water*
- *incense*
- *small altar*
- *bible*
- *candles (optional)*

The Doll:

Theoretically you could use any doll as long as you can visualize the person in the process. So if you can't make the doll or don't know of anyone who can you can always substitute something else. The reason I suggest making it is that there is an element of 'your' own heart that goes into making it that helps in the prayer process seem more real and helps you visualize what you are about to do. Photocopy or cut out the patterns in this book out and use them and if you need a wider margin to sew on you can cut make it larger by simply cutting an even width that is wider around the doll and clothes or enlarging it on your computer. My dolls are larger than those in this book because of the format allowed in printing I was unable to put the actual size in the book. They are available on my website for you to print however. You can also scan the pattern from the book into your computer and use the enlarge feature to increase your pattern size.

To make the doll you will need the following items:

- *1/3 yd. Muslin or some fabric (color choice is up to you)*
- *polyester stuffing*
- *1/3 yd. White cotton fabric for the gown. White is best as it represents our righteousness in Christ*
- *Personal items such as locks of hair, jewelry, or something of personal value to the one you are praying over.*
- *A picture of their face if you can get it*

Now pin your pattern to the fabric making sure that you cut two pieces at once. There should be enough to make a couple dolls. Cut out the doll.

- *Remove the pattern and sew around the doll leaving the area marked 'open' open.*
- *Snip the corners slightly so that they will turn inside out better.*
- *Then, once you've sown around the doll with a regular stitch I like to go back and zigzag it to make sure it doesn't fray and open.*
- *Turn the doll right side out and stuff it.*
- *Hand stitch the hole shut.*

(The reason I used muslin is that it is a very natural fabric and I felt it represented our dust from whence we came. Any fabric will do however and you can even buy no name brand flat sheets which are remarkably cheap compared to most fabrics.)

Warning: Do not make the doll with intentional blemishes like one leg missing or arm etc. Also do not make it 'gender' specific. There is no male or female in Christ Jesus. We are complete in Christ and so we will be thinking down that line of thought, okay? Good :)

The gown:

- *Cut the pattern out and lay the gown onto the fabric and pin it into place.*
- *Cut the gown out and choose the regular or the longer sleeved.*

- *Snip the collar area with 'tiny' snips to help it hem under and only turn the hem over once like a fold.*
- *Sew the collar hem.*
- *Next, hem the sleeves with a very small doubled hem by folding it over two times.*
- *Then sew the sides down and do the same type of hem to the bottom of the gown.*

Again, the reason we are using a white gown is to respect and represent the doll as a child of purity and Truth. One must be cautious to not take the wrong approach and establish negative energy into the doll or towards the doll. At no point and time should you feel as if you are overpowering someone or abusing them. If you feel aggressive toward the doll it is a sign that your heart is not ready to pray for the person you are attempting to help. Please go back to the meditation until you can proceed with the doll in a loving manner. Otherwise you are practicing Voodoo and no child of God should be doing that, right?

You can put personal items inside the doll if you like or sew them on afterward. Putting personal items into the doll would signify it as always being a certain person. If you wish to use the doll for multiple people, I suggest removable items on the outside of the doll.

The Cross:

In the REEDOO process I use a cloth cross to lay the person on to. I do this as I visualize them in Christ. To make the cross take some left over white fabric or whatever you have and hem it to make a cross. This can be two rectangle pieces the lay over each other and then the rope is used to form a special circle and I will show you how to do that in a minute. Remember, these are ONLY visual aids! It was through visualization that the worlds are formed and exist as we know them and it is our visualization of Him in us that leads us. Without a vision of Truth the people of God perish. We are going to visualize, visualize, visualize!

My cross is about 16 inches high. As long as it is at least a foot high you should be fine. You could make the cross out of felt for ease of construction and it would also lay nicely and adhere to any fabric surface.

The Blessing and Deliverance Process

I cannot stress enough the importance of making sure you don't have any anger or personal agendas in what you are doing. If you do, you are not praying(blessing) any more but cursing and practicing Voodoo. There is a method which I will include that allows you to pray for someone whom you are upset with as there are usually aspects to any frustrating relationship that are positive and the positive things can be built upon while the Holy Spirit works on your heart on the other issues through the meditation.

When we move by faith, things change. Fear is just faith in evil and if you fear God in a bad way it will not bless you at all. Real fear of God means that you respect Him/Truth. We don't serve who we fear. Fear present means we serve ourselves and are afraid of the person(s) who we think can 'take us out'. What we fear is soon to come upon us. When we are born again we are not given this spirit. This spirit is not of the Father. Fear fruits evil into your life because a demonic spirit has given you the understanding of fear. God is not the author of fear. God is faith itself. When He begins to reveal Himself to you it will be your response to what he has shown you through revelation that will produce fruit in your life and fear of evil will become a thing of the past like every other sin. Christians who don't understand fear just aren't mature enough yet so be patient, even with yourself, concerning all spiritual issues. We are all growing and if we don't move on what we've learned how can we continue to grow? How can God produce fruit in your life if you refuse to become fertile and receive the seed of Truth? This is why faith without works is dead and all the ceremonial aspects of this book are only meant to build your faith in what you are doing and seeing in your spirit. There isn't power in the doll or the little bits of fabric and string that hold it together. The power comes from the promises of God and from His word that whatsoever we bind on earth is bound in heaven and that if we ask anything according to His will He hears us! Brethren, use the instruments before you and move upon what you know is right.

Even so faith, if it hath not works, is dead, being alone.

James 2:17 (KJV)

And the prayer of faith shall save the sick, and the Lord shall raise him up; and if he have committed sins, they shall be forgiven him.

James 5:15 (KJV)

What if you never prayed? Would it do you any good to know all there is to know about deliverance or healing if you never use it? This is the power behind the dolls and the ceremony. You are moving by faith. You are calling things that are not as though they were! All you are doing is using visual aides to give you a hands on point of contact to transfer the power of God to the hurting person. If you turn around and place your faith in your visual aides you have defeated the purpose and created a new religion and a cult! Don't let that happen to you! It is the temptation of the flesh to accredit power to things, and ceremonies tend to enhance the flesh when done with pride. In reality the only way that God's Spirit will move is by faith because He is Faith and He doesn't move according to anyone's wrong thoughts or motives. We see in Hebrews that faith is the very essence of what we hope for and the evidence of what is not yet seen. You have to 'see' it in your minds eye before you see it in matter. This is how God created the world and how you will recreate the world around you.

Now faith is the substance of things hoped for, the evidence of things not seen.
Heb 11:1 (KJV)

You cannot be pleasant unto the Father without believing Him and what He says. You can't come to God and call Him a liar, hate the Truth, and then expect to be at One with Him and get a great big hug of approval.

But without faith it is impossible to please him: for he that cometh to God must believe that he is, and that he is a rewarder of them that diligently seek him.
Heb 11:5-6 (KJV)

There are some other things you can also use in your blessing ceremonies. I suggest that you only use those that have a revelational meaning to you and you may discover more than I have put here. I would love to hear what you learn so that I too may be blessed! You can also share your experiences and ideas on the forum connected to the website and bless others.

If you understand the power of anointing oil then use the oil. If you grasp the meaning of holy water, use holy water. I will give a brief breakdown of the things that God has shown me and perhaps it will also bless you. God is infinite and so when you follow Him you will find infinite ways of doing things!

REEDOO is so flexible. You can create your prayer circle by simply sitting on the floor or on your bed or some place comfortable and doing a formal REEDOO session or you can skip the cross and the string and just do a very informal session by holding the doll as you walk around proclaiming the Truth over it, anointing it with oil etc, as the Holy Spirit leads. No two prayer sessions need to be alike as no two situations concerning a person in need will be the same.

Here is an example of a basic REEDOO session and what I suggest when you do the first session on a new person or for yourself for the first time is that give the doll the identity of the person you are praying for.

Example of a very basic REEDOO session:

1. Begin with a request. "Father I ask in the name of Jesus that your Holy Spirit will lead this blessings ceremony and that your angels would carry out Your words that I speak and that none of them would fall to the ground."

2. Lay out the cross on the floor or bed area where you will be standing or sitting. Do this while holding the doll or keeping it near you and say, "This cross represents your only begotten Son, Jesus Christ."

3. Take the string and make a circle around yourself, the doll ,and the cross and say, "This is the circle of Truth. There is nothing outside of this circle and within this circle only the Truth remains. Hence we are in Christ within the Truth and only that which is in this circle is Real."

4. Hold the doll firmly and seriously and establish who it represents to your understanding. Say something like, "I now proclaim this doll to represent the spirit, soul, and body of (say the name of the person the doll represents).

5. Lay the doll onto the cross and say, "(name of doll) is in Christ Jesus. All things are new. I henceforth know this person no longer after their flesh".

6. Take some anointing oil that has already been prayed over (read below for more information) and place some on the dolls forehead and say while visualizing them, "You are the anointed of God. I sanctify and consecrate you in the name of Jesus. By faith I declare you set apart unto God, holy, and without blame in Christ Jesus"

7. Begin to profess the Truth over them, do a deliverance, or whatever the Lord lays on your heart. I will cover effective deliverance techniques after I explain group ceremonies.

8. If you say something that wasn't right and you catch it, say, " I repent or recant and rebuke that in Jesus name". You can also command it to fall to the ground in Jesus name or return it to the unclean spirit that sent you that bad information!

9. After you are done blessing, close the ceremony with the Word or informally if you are walking around holding the doll praying in tongues for example. Just lay the doll down respectfully. If you are doing a more formal setting you can close with an Amen. Which means, "it is so". You have just bound what you said or signed and sealed it.

Some of the other items you might want to use in a blessing ceremony may be water you have prayed over, oil, or even burn incense to represent the sweet savor of the prayers you are about to offer to the Lord. And you may light candles if you do it safely and for the right reasons but don't do it to 'feel' spiritual. You want to move from your understanding and for the right reasons in all that you do to avoid any kind of negative reaction. Let the Holy Spirit lead you for however long it takes and move according to what you see in your spirit.

Try to practice it more formally only when you know you won't be interrupted by phone calls, small children, or office calls. You don't want to put yourself into an overwhelming situation where you will get angry for having to give your attention to something else.

"Who has time for all this?", I hear you asking. Well, for one, you can stop going to those dead Wednesday night prayer meetings. Instead, call some friends and make it a REEDOO night at your house and watch the power of God unleash!

The Deliverance Process:

The aspects of deliverance commands in REEDOO is very important and often the heart of the REEDOO session. Therefore we will cover the basic deliverance commands in this section of the book.

What is deliverance? Deliverance is a noun. That means that it is something 'tangible'. When a person is truly saved from something that is trying to destroy one, this is a tangible thing! It is nice to know that you are making a tangible difference in the lives of others when using the REEDOO method.

The word deliverance means:

1. **an act or instance of delivering.**
2. **salvation.**
3. **liberation.**
4. **a thought or judgment expressed; a formal or authoritative pronouncement.**

To receive liberation from unclean spirits is the very point and reason to have or do a deliverance. To understand freedom from unclean spirits, it helps if one first understands the aspect of 'entanglement'. Comprehending how and why the unclean spirit can enter or access one's own spirit is paramount in becoming free.

Most deliverance ministries have it wrong. They teach you to battle in an ignorant and arrogant way--- actually in your flesh. They teach you to come from a place of pride and duke it out with evil spirits. This is extremely damaging theology to all involved in that kind of process. Often people lose their lives due to this kind of thinking. These ministers and pushers of this theology speak great swelling words from pride but if you go visit or interview the people they have 'helped' you will find greater cripples than when those people first asked for deliverance! My question is, was that real deliverance? No! Absolutely not and I could right an entire volume on why but for now lets look at real deliverance.

True deliverance is when God/Truth overcomes the devils/lies in your life. The Truth alone sets us free. In the bible we see Jesus who is called the 'Spirit of Truth' casting out unclean spirits with his words and healing people. This is what we will be doing but I don't want you to take it lightly. I do not advise anyone to cast devils out of another person without seeking God on the matter first. The reason? You can easily make a situation worse for someone by doing such. If that person is not repentant they can be entered even stronger by demonic spirits and if you torment devils in their lives these people often feel that torment as if it were them and their bodies will begin to hurt as you come against the unclean spirits in them because they have become bound to the spirit behind the scene. I know this is hard to hear, but it is true. When we go to sleep consciously it is because their minds arose and awoke in us, and it is no longer you that lives, but them.

Just look out how our minds work. If you don't want to hear a particular truth and someone forces that truth down your throat, you immediately put up a taller wall of lies with all the necessary excuses and make a vow to not let that happen to you again. You 'harden' your heart, in other words. This allows more dark energy to enter because you have sunk in frequency by ignoring the Truth that you once had. This has made your spirit harder to access with the Truth and is also the reason that we must seek to not speak Truth to dull ears and why Jesus Himself would only speak in parables to those who couldn't hear the plain truth. He really cared for them and didn't want to make their situations worse than they already were and said that he came not to condemn. We must also do exactly what He did and do what is best for others.

In deliverance, and I'm talking about the kind where the person is standing in front of you, you will never be able to get anyone to separate from a devil that they love. Therefore, if a person thinks that their pride is them and does not seek to separate, how can you cast out that demon? This is the reason that many cannot get free from illnesses. They have become the unclean spirits in their lives and you would have to cast out that persons own spirit with the devils in order to deliver them! This is the reason why many are bound. True repentance is the only true separation from demonic entities.

Devils are basically lies. There are many and I mean MANY religious liars out there who lie about the deliverance process and salvation. They speak only the amount of truth that they must in order to get the ego food their sick souls desire. These voices that speak lies are devils behind the scene who love positions of importance and this world. These are the unclean spirits that Jesus sent away. You will not be able to see them clearly in others until you honestly seek separation from lies in your own life. Until you do, you will be conned on a continual basis and drawn to the ones in others that you already follow in you.

There is an untimely and unseasonable time for deliverance to occur. When someone is not willing to see the Truth about their particular illness or situation it is not time to do a deliverance. Seek the Father on every person(s) that you are about to pray for and He will guide you in it. Everything that we do must be done in a way that helps the person the most and not any two people are the same.

Jesus told a woman who had sinned and was ill as a result of it that if she continued to sin (move upon wrong thinking) an even stronger and worse spirits(voices) would come to her. We are just the same way. The best way to jump out of the frying pan into the fire is to seek to rid one's self of faults but only so you can become perfectly wicked. The arrogant mind is always in pursuit of its own state and idea of perfection and glory. Therefore, be wise and look at the real picture. Is the person you are praying for ready for deliverance? Are they ready to repent? Do you see honest humility and true heart felt seeking of God? If they are not, and you know it, you can pray for their heart to be moved to repentance and stick to those kinds of phrases instead of the ones I am about to share on deliverances.

Remember, sending positive energy is sending angels, negative energy is any kind of thought or emotion that is not of God and will send people unclean spirits. Anger, pride, lust, envy, greed, and such things are of the devil and not of God and will send LF into the person you are thinking about. Be wise and sense where you are coming from when you seek to help another soul and then move according to what you hear in you. If you are coming from the right place in your heart you will hear correctly. Forgive yourself for mistakes and you will be able to forgive others as well.

As I share some commands and concepts that you can use to help others, I suggest that you only use the ones that command devils to leave when you know the person is ready for them to do so but you may find yourself moved to speak the commands as you are in the middle of a REEDOO session. I would follow my heart. If the heart is set on really blessing, you will be correct in what you do.

There really are only several basic commands that I use. You may have others that you like to use that God has shown you. Remember, when we move from the Holy Spirit, we are Him in the earth. He has creation powers and all knees bow to the name of Jesus. That word is deeper than just syllables and changing it to Yeshua or Allah makes no difference. Our words are just sounds. It is the intent in the heart/spirit that emits correct frequency and words only express thought. You could say any word as long as your understanding was aligned with an understanding of Truth and it would mean what you thought. Religious people have trouble because they are pre-programmed and most do not move from understanding which is why they argue all the time and love to debate. They really don't have anything but empty sounds which they use to shoot each other with while they move from the spirit of pride.

Deliverance Commands:

(When speaking to an unclean spirit)

1. "I destroy (over ride, break, come against) your spirit (energy, power, presence) in Jesus name."

You are placing God's authority against the devils, verbally. Speaking verbally transmits vibrations. If you are coming from the right place in you, those vibrations will not return void!

2. "I bind (adjure, arrest, handcuff, capture) you in Jesus name."

This is important because you are in effect 'arresting' the spirit that is causing the problem. Remember, whatever you bind on earth is bound in heaven. That means that HF overrules LF. Now that you have arrested the villain. What do you do with a felon? We are going to read the spirit its rights and put it away.

3. "In Jesus name I loose (remove, break, pull) you from this body and I command you to leave (go to your grave, into the earth, to the pit,) in Jesus name."

Or you can pick a destination. You can send them into the earth, to their grave, to the pit, the moon, or where ever the Holy Spirit impresses you to send them. You are in control of them but it is not in an arrogant way. You honestly want what is best for all spirits concerned, even the unclean ones.

*Unclean spirits are going to be judged after the thousand year reign when death, hell, and the sea give up the dead (Rev. 20:13). Therefore, realize that their judgment day is coming and **never** seek 'revenge' against any spirit. To do so is an act of pride and an LF thought and emotion and it would mean that you are moving from an unclean spirit in yourself to aid someone else who is being victimized by an unclean spirit which is just not going to work and also means you are working in conjunction with them which is what 'all' prideful deliverance ministers are really doing! Horrible to say the least!*

Instead, seek the Father's face on how to deal with the spirit. Send it to a destination that is given to you and do it without remorse or joy. Be emotionless in that action. (In my seminars and conferences I teach you how to confront spirits of the dead and undead and how not to get overcome in the deliverance process.)

Other things that you can do is to ask the angels to be present around the person you are praying for. Envision them coming and standing around the person or over the person. Reach out your hand and envision touching their aura. You can run your hand over the shape of the person in your minds eye. I did this once for several hours while praying in tongues for a person and they nearly freaked out because they said that they felt a fuzzy sensation all over their head! They could feel the positive energy of God flowing into them! See it and believe it and it will be.

Also, become observant and really watch what your mouth sends out. Our bodies are shaped, molded, and guided by our mouths. We also shape the lives of others and the bible tells us that our bodies and lives are guided by our mouths and that our religion is in vain or pointless if our mouths do not speak the truth that we have been shown.

(Do the above three in succession as listed to stop demonic activity in your life or others.)

Other commands:

4. "I command the liver (body parts, etc.) to function normally in Jesus name."

I have had extreme success in commanding the flesh to obey. You have full authority in Christ to come against the works of the devil. One of those works is sickness. Commanding a leg to grow, blood to return to normal, circulation systems to function, brains to function, etc. is easy for the Holy Spirit to do. Let the Holy Spirit guide you in what you command and make sure it is all done in Jesus name.

Jesus is in you. It is no longer you that lives, but Christ within you. It is Him doing the work so there is no reason to wonder if you can make it work...it isn't you doing the work! This is very important to understand. The more you see that, the stronger your faith will grow and you will not be speaking anymore, but Christ in you will do the talking!

5. "I rebuke you devil in Jesus name. Come out of this person and leave in Jesus name."

This is a very affective short statement. I have found that it is not in the best interest in all present to let emotions rise and shouting to occur when doing a deliverance. Whilst screaming, your own behavior suggests a spirit of fear which will only fuel the unclean spirits grip on the person you are praying for and cause emotional trauma. Instead, speak like you mean it, because you do, but do so firmly, without fear, and in full confidence. It is faith that moves mountains, not noise. Visualize everything you are doing and saying and realize that the power of God is moving through you and you are not the source of it and He will perform the work. Therefore, if you speak from a mind other than His, nothing will happen and you are not in control of Him, He controls you. Be prepared for nothing to happen as well. Many healings take time to occur. Let everything be what it is and do not struggle in pride (wrong spirit) to make things happen. Let the outcome be what it is and don't let it bother you. Just focus on the Holy Spirit and follow as best you can.

The ego tends to want to identify with what one does and to also take credit or discredit. It measures its 'self' by what it considers a success, meaning that it got what it wanted. However, put some common sense against it and it will fold. For instance, if you successfully cure a person who would have repented otherwise and they die later on and go to hell, was that a success? Don't assume you know anything and especially not everything. Just follow the Holy Spirit and leave the outcomes to Him.

REEDOO offers some relief during some of the common stresses experienced in deliverance ministry as you do not have to deal with the persons noise, interruptions, and spirits directly that you are delivering. This is in some ways advantageous in that you can smoothly intercept and as you become more adept at hearing from the Holy Spirit and moving from Him you will be able to command in perfect unison with Him and your words will change the lives of many.

6. "The blood of Jesus"

You can do what is commonly referred to as 'pleading the blood of Jesus' over someone. To do this you begin by visualizing the blood of Jesus. Perhaps it is the blood coming from his thorny crowns. See the crowns piercing his skull and the blood running down his face. This blood is sacred, sinless, and pure. All who believe into Jesus' life and death and who have given their lives to Him (His life and death) are the saved. Know that that blood cleanses us from sin and that He died for the whole world.

Next, visualize the person you are praying for and let the blood from Jesus wash down over the person you are praying for. You can place them at the foot of the cross and let Jesus' blood begin to cleanse them. Demons 'hate' this! Trust me...it works! You can also put the blood of Jesus into the unclean spirits mouth and anywhere on them and they will scream and despise the purity of Jesus.

Jesus rebuked devils and people were healed. You can do this too because Jesus is in you. We are even commanded to do so. I think that deliverance ministry is perhaps one of the most misused and lost ministries out there. Most are fighting the figments of their imaginations and moving from unclean spirits in the process and hurting others as well as themselves.

Without understanding what do we have to move from? Therefore, with all thy getting....get understanding because without it any devil can lead you anywhere it wants as long as your mind is in the dark..

If you live in the dark the darkness lives through you. The fruits of darkness are sickness and death, confusion and futility. Just as a plant dies from lack of sunshine, so will you in both spirit and body if you are separated from the Light.

Every human being needs exactly what you need to live. We are all of Him. Realize then that what is truly good for you is truly good for someone else. What truly blessed your life, also blesses others and often we hate what is truly good for us.

Patience with our fellow man needs to start in our own lives and forgiveness must begin in you first before you can ever practice it upon another soul.

Whether we like it or not we practice what we believe....even if what we believe is wrong and so we cannot help be lost in all the areas where we do not have the Truth in our hearts to move from and what you practice in your own life upon yourself you will automatically practice upon others. It is impossible to truly love (overlook, be patient, or kind) someone else unless you first treat your own spirit with the same courtesy.

Preparing items for use

Items you may use or need:

- **Oil** *(Olive oil, cooking oil, or fragrance oil ....home made fragrance oils are also great)*
- **Water**
- **Incense**
- **Bible**
- **Crucifix or a cross** *(a cross necklace also works well and can be left around the dolls neck)*
- **7 White Tea Light Candles and holders** ....*(and something to light them with)*
- **8-12' of white butchers twine, string, or small rope**

(Hints: Use neat bottles you find lying around like small seasoning bottles etc. Also, for the water I like to use something I can put my fingers into and then flick my fingers. Something with a wide mouth to it that seals well works great.)

Oil:

Oil was used in the bible to consecrate an item or person unto God. We are the sons of God. We are set apart and an holy priesthood. There are no male or female spirits. We are all one in Him and of One body. Jesus' body isn't male on one side and female on the other! What? Did the revelations of God come to you men only or did it come to us women too? Do we have a right to move from the Holy Spirit as well as you? Not only do we have a right but an obligation to obey the Lord. Mistranslations and interpretations have done much damage to the body of Christ. Any role a man can do a woman can too because it isn't us that is moving but the Holy Spirit. There is neither male nor female in Christ.

You can use any kind of cooking oil. There are some companies that offer fragrance oils. Olive oil is also fine and works well. I take a small container of oil and hold it while I pray in tongues, infusing the HF from the Holy Spirit into it. This is the 'essence' of God. You can also say, "I put the essence of God in this oil in Jesus name" because that is what you are doing when you hold it and pray. You are believing that God's Energy is permeating it and it really is so it isn't as if you have to make it happen. Visualize it happening. Your are creating from the Holy Spirit and you must visualize it!

Use this oil in ceremonies and in real life. The longer you hold it the more faith you will have towards it when you use it. It is sacred. God is in it. The power behind it is the visualization of what it is and what it is doing. You are creating by the power of the Holy Spirit that is moving in you. This is what He does in and through us and how His will is brought forth in the earth.

You can anoint areas on the doll that represent sicknesses on the person's body. What you are saying is, 'this part that the devils are trying to destroy is consecrated and sacred ground!'. Healing can happen just from a strong visualization of that alone!

And thou shalt put them upon Aaron thy brother, and his sons with him; and shalt anoint them, and consecrate them, and sanctify them, that they may minister unto me in the priest's office. ***Ex 28:41 (KJV)***

We are also told to anoint the sick with oil and they will recover after supplication and prayer is made by a person who is close to God's heart. James 5:14-15 (KJV)

Water:

Water represents the Spirit of God. Put some water in a container and breathe into it. Say, "this is the breathe of God" breathe again into the water and say, "the Spirit of God is in this water". Then in the ceremony sprinkle the water onto the person when you feel something blocking the healing or deliverance. Visualize light entering the body and removing darkness. See devils fleeing as you sprinkle the doll with the water. Envision the person you are helping. See their energy level rising, their health returning, and their souls crying out to the Father to hear and know the Truth.

Incense:

You can burn incense and it will mean more if you understand why you are doing it. Incense represents that which is pleasant to God and represents your full persuasion that you believe that God is hearing you. The veil was torn upon Jesus' death and we have full access to the Father to offer our prayers up as a sweet smell to Him. The prayers that are pleasing to God are only the prayers that are made in faith which will be what you are doing.

For incense you can get fancy and buy an actual swinging incense holder or you can just light a good smelling candle or incense stick. You can see the process in the scripture below. God has mercy upon you if you pray from a sincere heart and it pleases Him that you are seeking the Truth in your heart.

They sell incense sticks and cones which burn and are relatively inexpensive and widely accessible to the public. Make sure that you use safety when lighting any candles or incense as you don't want people to be reaching across an open flame and setting themselves on fire. Use wisdom and realize that these items simply represent thought that creates matter. Of themselves a candle, oil, and water, etc. don't do anything but they only help you visualize what is occurring in the spirit realm. Swinging an incense holder would be a great job for a someone who is a little shy in a group setting. They could actively participate but be sort of aloof at the same time by circling the table with the mobile incense holder, supporting the prayers of their brethren, praying in tongues as they swing the holder.

And he shall take a censer full of burning coals of fire from off the altar before the LORD, and his hands full of sweet incense beaten small, and bring it within the vail: 13 And he shall put the incense upon the fire before the LORD, that the cloud of the incense may cover the mercy seat that is upon the testimony, that he die not:

Lev 16:12-13 (KJV)

Let my prayer be set forth before thee as incense; and the lifting up of my hands as the evening sacrifice.   Psalms 141:2 (KJV)

.

And the smoke of the incense, which came with the prayers of the saints, ascended up before God out of the angel's hand.
Rev 8:4 (KJV)

Candles:

I suggest white candles and seven of them to represent the seven energy points and aspects of God's own Spirit. What I like to do is place seven candle holders (small ones) around the doll and light them in order of their energy points and claim the churches for Jesus. Speaking the Word over each and every aspect of the person you are praying for. I usually only use this method when I do group prayer or if someone is really sick. Be careful using candles in the circle and don't do it on a flammable surface. Tea light candles work well but be careful if you do group ceremonies not to catch someone's sleeve on fire!

These things saith he that hath the seven Spirits of God, ……….Rev 3:1 (KJV)

God's Spirit has seven aspects. We have seven too as we are made in His image. Remember, He is the All Spirit God. Therefore, if you want to recognize this aspect in your ceremony you could light each candle and bless each energy point according to their name in Revelations. Remember, there are the seven aspects to your spirit. If a sin blocks one of these energy points or it becomes lowered in frequency and no longer receives any HF, it will begin to die. It is covered extensively in my book "How to Be a Spiritual

Christian". Also, I use white candles to represent purity in spirit.

Every aspect of this ceremony is done to aide in visualization of what is going on in the spirit realm. If you do all this from a carnal mindset and just enjoy feeling royally spiritual and powerful, you will fail at helping anyone and become the next foolish witch or sorcerer. Cleansing your heart before you touch anything is a must! Do the meditation and Communion daily. Fasting doesn't hurt either. Especially right before a group ceremony as they are more intense.

Bible:

A small bible is very efficient used in dealing with unclean spirits and LF. It represents all HF thoughts. You are in effect telling disembodied spirits that you mean business!

To use it you can press the doll with it or place the bible on the doll. Also, you can use it to point or touch the doll in specific places while commanding out demonic spirits. What this represents is your faith in God's Words and His thoughts and ways. You are openly placing your trust in Him and showing your confidence in Good over evil, Right over wrong, and Truth over lies. Take your bible and place it directly against the lies of the enemy.... directly against the evil things the demons are trying to do to harm this person. In essence you are saying, "I believe God and not you, devil!" and that is faith.

The bible is taught to most Christians as the Inspired Word of God and that if they move an 'a' round or forget a period where it was meant to be that their names will be blotted out of the Book of Life. Although this creates difficulty in receiving revelations from the Holy Spirit, it does set a solid *faith that the Bible is God and so in deliverances and prayers the amount of faith in holding a bible over an evil spirit is profoundly strong. Us this aspect wisely in group sessions and let all bring their bibles into the circle if they desire.*

Crucifix:

You already have the doll on a cross. You may also place a cross on the doll. This can represent several things to your understanding. One of them is that you are placing your faith in what Jesus did for all of us on the cross right into the face of a devil that is trying to make a person sick. You direct this visualization of Christ, His blood, and the resurrection power right on the individual's energy points and bringing the power of God against the disembodied spirits that are attacking them. The crucifix is a very well known powerful weapon against dark energy and demons HATE it! A powerful place to use it is on the 6th energy point or what some call your third eye. This is the direct line or highway/window into your soul. Often people who are touched on the forehead pass out. Some call it slain in the spirit. You can actually cause yourself to fall out too. You may get a feeling that you are about to during mediation at times.

Take your time and focus upon what you are doing in REEDOO and move from what you understand. Keep seeking God and asking Him for better ways and see what He shows you. It is better to do one thing right than 20 in a sloppy confused manner. Simple moments of laying hands on the doll and just saying, "I bless you in Jesus name", from the bottom of a well heart can go a long way to the healing and regeneration of another soul.

Please don't take this too far and make it into witchcraft; the art of controlling someone else. We are in this to bless people, not curse them or try to rule over anyone.

Altar:

Okay, before you get all up in your religious spirit and scream...witchcraft! I knew it! I would like to point out to you that your church has an altar. They give an altar call at nearly every service I've ever been too. You know, where you come to the front and kneel at a little altar and pray? Well we are going to make a useable work surface so we don't set anything on fire or hurt ourselves and others and I'm going to call it an altar because it is where we are going to be praying at, just like at church. The table/alter will be discussed in more detail in the next chapter but is an integral part of REEDOO.

It may not seem relevant here but I want to remind everyone of the scientific evidence of sending positive energy to plants. In studies it has been proven that plants grown under glass in controlled settings would grow differently depending on the thoughts that people would send to them. A person would speak loving caring words to one set of plants and then the next set would be cursed. The results? The blessed plants flourished and the cursed ones were stunted! We emit energy and we send it. Lets make sure we are sending 'positive' energy to others.

Group Sessions

REEDOO in group sessions is a bit different as you have others present in the circle and the doll must be able to be accessed by everyone. Also, everyone present needs a basic understanding of what they are going to do and how REEDOO works. Like I mentioned before, what I chose to do was make a round table to express unity and it also makes it equally easy for everyone to access the altar and the items on the table. We are all going to commence our prayers here at this round table. I also found it necessary to have at least two and sometimes three people to act as elders in the group because you need a way to monitor the group and keep the prayer circle going.

You need at least two people who can discern if words are coming from devils or the Holy Spirit during the ceremony and these individuals must also have enough grace to politely correct and patiently teach others. This isn't as easy as it sounds. Usually the most arrogant want to be great 'leaders' and will get offended when you put anyone else but them in charge. Do not let this intimidate you and cause you to put them in charge. It will end in disaster if you do. There are also group manners which we will discuss and I will put forth a set of rules that seem to work well for us. **I will also put a thread for this process on Bread and Wine Ministries forum. If you learn anything new that could bless the group or you just want to testify how REEDOO has changed your life, please feel free to post it. We would love to hear how REEDOO is changing lives around the world.**

The Table:

I made my own table but what you can do is purchase one of those cheap circle tables that they sell for round end tables. Cover it with one of the covers that they sell for them. White is nice but will stain and so I also suggest a round glass top to go on top of the table. You can leave a permanent cross under the glass and the whole thing is candle safe, oil proof, and wipes up easily. You can also hot glue the candle holders to the glass for safety if you want to. The only draw back is that those particular tables tend to be a bit wobbly which is why I chose to make my own.

Remember, you can do REEDOO by simply carry the doll around praying in tongues or you can do a full blown ceremony with a group and gowns to boot! It is entirely flexible. The central point of the process is your heart praying for others and having a visual aid and point of contact.

In group REEDOO we discovered that you need to elect a point man and two wing men (right and left). The point man is the first person who directs the group and if he/she needs to step out of the circle, the right one steps into his/her place and then the left one steps up if the right one steps out.

The point man should be one who is able to discern spirit entities and know the character of God as they will have to make decisions as to whether or not something that was said came from the right source. The gift of discernment is crucial for the elders. They must be able to tell when a demon is speaking or the Holy Spirit. They aren't in charge of who does what in the group but are simply an overseer of what is said and 'felt' in order to keep it a blessing ceremony and not a cursing one. Each member of the group needs to know the 'rules' before they take part of the ceremony and don't let a person who is moving from the wrong motivation into the group in a way that would hurt people. There are ways to include those who are not as aware of which spirit they are moving from and still have a great session without hurting anyone's feelings. The gift of wisdom will help you in this matter.

Group Manners:

It must be explained to your group or any new person joining that the circle is about helping people. It is not a place to prove anything to anyone. Pride needs to be chucked at the door! You must be prepared to be questioned and realize that not one person is going to get it right all the time and that we are all here to help people and we often just simply misunderstand each other and need help to understand. This meeting is about helping others.

Try and get them to understand that everyone has wrong thinking that they move from and so odds are that we all at some point will say something out of line and it will get noticed. And it is highly possible that you will be right on track and simply misunderstood or misinterpreted by another member. **Questioning the speaker is an act of safety for the group and the person being prayed over and it is not to be used as personal elevation!** If a person has a severe problem with criticism then suggest to them that they do more simple things like just say, "bless you in Jesus name", or to pray in tongues quietly, lay hands on the doll while doing so or even keep their hands aimed at the doll while praying gently in the background. Also, let them know that if the point man thinks that pouring the entire bottle of anointing oil on a table lit with candles isn't a good idea unless you want a barbeque, please be ready for some gentle reprisal. Even the point man can be questioned in the circle. Why? Everyone is accessed by LF and we all want this to work! Getting everyone on the same page is *crucial to successful REEDOO.*

Let each person speak as they are moved by the Holy Spirit. No two should be talking over the other or in competition and all must reverence the Holy Spirit as He moves. If a person says something from the wrong spirit or that another person doesn't think is right they may say, "Clarification please"...the please must be included and spoken in a gentle manner.

The statement that was questioned then returns to the one who spoke it and they have a chance to clarify it or move on. If they realize they spoke from the wrong spirit or do not wish to be confronted, they may say, "I recant". If they feel strongly about what they said and wish to clarify they may do so or they may say, "pass" and everyone will simply overlook the statement, commit it to God, and go on without repeating that statement again. If the person who made the statement decides to clarify it and it is still an LF one or one not understood it may once again be returned to the speaker. Only really serious things need to be clarified. The group must be willing to allow a margin of error for humanities sake and seek to not shut down the REEDOO session over small issues or wording and such. The point man is in charge as far as how far the clarification process goes. If it becomes disruptive they may adjourn the circle by saying, "the circle is broken" because a spirit of discord has entered it and there is no discord in Truth. Everyone must stop to minister to those with hurt feelings till all is well and only then can they come back into agreement and the process began again. If they cannot, the session is over and the next group must be more in accordance with the Truth. WARNING! If someone gets there feelings hurt they most likely will avoid group REEDOO. We don't want anyone to stop, so avoid confrontations as much as possible. God listens to wrong prayers all day long and His grace covers us quite easily. Only confront serious issues that will harm the group or the person being prayed for.

All emotions should be as positive as humanly possible. Let each member know that they can step out of the circle for any reason without shame. If they need to use the restroom, blow their nose, or need a moment to forgive someone, the group must not condemn it. If the point man sees that a negative spirit has entered the group and even one or two members have become angry, mocking, or cruel the ceremony **must** *be temporarily or permanently halted. The situation must be restored and that spirit gone before the meeting continues. A dark spirit also often can be commanded out silently by the leader in the name of Jesus without making a scene. Don't forget that if tensions begin to mount, that you can break for snacks and drinks and then restarted on a more positive note with loving heart felt ideas or bits of wisdom and direction upon the next session. Ask others what the Holy Spirit is showing them before you begin and it will help the whole group stir up the gifts in them. Be positive, kind, and open. Also, if one person that you are praying over is causing tension upon the group you can place a new subject into the circle and often this will lighten the groups heart to begin again.*

If spirits send in a disruptive member who repeats an offense or seems to systematically destroy the group, that person must not be invited to the next session and privately disciplined by at least two people. Odds are if you do that they will not return to the church again so don't be cruel. How would you like to be treated? This will answer all your questions in dealing with others. What is really good for them is also good for you. Don't be a hypocrite. Receive what you also give out.

Let everyone in the group know a week in advance of a ceremony. You can use white robes if you like to represent unity and purity in Christ. But keep things light, fun, and positive. Don't get overly religious or dark and judgmental. Keeping the groups small of about 6 or 8 until you get the hang of it will help to keep things flowing smoothly as well and then add new members at a gradual pace unless the Holy Spirit directs otherwise.

The Group Ceremony:

Items needed:

- **round table with cross**
- **30+' of cotton rope**
- **robes for the members (white)-totally optional...teens love it!**
- **Blessing items>Oil, Water, Bibles, Incense candles, matches or a lighter, doll(s)etc.**

If you are planning on doing this in your church I suggest a mandatory class that newbies must attend before they can practice REEDOO. Have someone teach the class on a regular basis and then place that person into a circle that best fits their character. Newbies will be able to 'get their feet wet' in class before entering a group. After they finish the class you could give them a robe and certificate upon completion and appoint them their first session.

Don't forget to give a weeks notice or at least a few days prior to any REEDOO session. This notice should come with names of people you will be praying for just in case there is someone on the list that they have problems dealing with. It gives the person a chance to get their ducks in a row and either bow out or face up to the truth in their heart concerning the person(s) being placed into the circle. Also, you can announce on a sheet who is in which REEDOO group. This will help discourage members from coming against each other and gives them time to prepare for the session.,

If anyone in the group has hurt feelings, unforgiveness, or animosity towards the person being ministered to or to someone else in the group they need to leave the group or be ministered to first until they can find a way to enter the circle without anger, animosity, jealousy, or pride towards an individual. If they are prone to anger outbursts, etc. perhaps they can do more preset phrases things like plead the blood of Jesus over the person, etc. Explain that in the teaching sessions that often 'less is more'. If the group lets dark energy in, the devil won and they just royally lost and got their butts whooped! Get it through to them that this is war and that the devil wants the circle to end. Will we oblige him or will we count the cost to our pride and do what is right and keep the circle alive for Jesus? All for One(God) and One(God) for all.

Also, it is often wise to keep the 'deep' phrases and confessions to yourself if no one else understands it and you know they don't. Don't tempt others to fight. Tell the group to stick to more well known things like blessings, tongues, pleading the blood of Jesus, etc. at first until they get a good feel of REEDOO. Let them know that they can present their thoughts before hand to the group if they are thinking of prayer certain phrases that are questionable and that they can discuss any issues that bother them or upset them after the meeting. Otherwise it will end quickly in theological debate! Devil's love to do this! For the groups sake tell them to keep things simple and positive and the name of the game is ….."don't let the devil in the circle!"

The Session:

- *Have all the members gather around the little table. Ask the Holy Spirit to bless and angels to be present.*

- *Verbally proclaim who the doll represents.*

- *Next, place the doll into Christ by saying something like, "(name) is in Christ Jesus. It is no longer (name) that lives but Christ Jesus. Place the doll onto the cross.*

- *Then the point man must take the cotton rope and make a circle around everyone while saying something like, "This circle represents the Truth. It is the beginning and the end and nothing is outside of the Truth. We are all one in Christ."*

- *(Optional): The candles are then lit in order of the churches, named, blessed, and proclaimed as belonging to the Father and made in His image. This can be done by any of the elders, just make sure you know who is going to do it to avoid confusion, giggling, etc.*

- *The point man or incense holder then lights the incense and says, "This represents our prayers. May they be pleasing and acceptable to You Heavenly Father."*

- *Next, the point man needs to step back and the group can either hold hands of pray in accordance saying "come Holy Spirit, we welcome you. Fill us with power from on High" until a stirring comes forth from an individual. Help them realize that there is no need to rush. Wait and be filled. This will feel like warm electricity washing over you. Let them anxiously, expectantly wait, and seek. Tell them what it feels like and they will envision His presence and their faith will move the Father's heart. Then, once a person is moved by the Father, the blessings begin to commence as the Holy Spirit directs using the items on the table as the individual feel prompted by the Holy Spirit.*

- *Keep moving and praying until you feel the answer has come or someone 'breaks the circle and lets a devil in' (see definition for broken circle). Don't get angry that it happened. The point man/person(s) must immediately seek wisdom to fix the situation. Also, you can beseech the group to pray for an answer to continue. No lone rangers allowed in this group!*

- *People can come and go out of the circle so long as the rhythm is not interfered with and positive energy is abounding. Negative energy is what you must avoid in the circle. As soon as it is felt, the interception process is to be stopped immediately. This is why we must avoid unnecessary confrontations at all costs.*

- *The point man needs to be sensitive to the Holy Spirit and move to the next doll/person when prompted. They also must be able to sort of 'guide' the ship along but not interfere or get an emotional high from the position.*

Broken Circle:

A circle is broken once strong negative energy is present in it. As we are human and have LF thoughts in and around us on a consistent basis, there will always be a measure of sin in us but strong, dangerous levels can do a lot of damage.....High levels of doubt, hate, anger, rage, resentment, jealousy, bitter envy, etc. are not acceptable as then your group is practicing witchcraft and voodoo. Please realize the severity of the matter and proceed with awareness and respect.

Blessing the Churches/Energy points and name definitions:

Here is a quick reference guide for the pronunciation of names and definitions. Also, I have included a sample blessing that you could use. Please realize that if something doesn't get spoken over, the world will go on. Be respectful but not strict or hateful and this will allow the Holy Spirit to move.

As long as you keep the meeting positive. You can include and exclude things as everyone sees fit. After all, people have been having prayer meetings in churches for years. The power of the meeting is that you are all in 'one accord', one mind, and one effort. Fasting in unison helps too and the same driving desire to see lives changed is powerful stuff!

- *Ephesus* > *(ef´ə səs)* > **first desirable**
- *Symrna* > *(smûr´nə)* > **bitter affliction**
- *Pergamum* > *(pûr´gə məm)* > **earthly heights**
- *Thyatira* > *(thī´ə tī´rə)* > **continual sacrifice**
- *Sardis* > *(sär´dis)* > **prince of joy**
- *Philadelphia* > *(fil´ə del´fē ə)* > **brotherly love**
- *Laodicea* > *(lā od´ə sē´ə, lā´ə də-)* > **people's opinion or people judged**

(These names could be engraved into the table or under the glass along with their meanings.)

Sample of positive confessions over the energy points:

- *"Ephesus, you have found the Truth*
- *Symnra, you have suffered for the Truth*
- *Pergamum, you have resisted lies*
- *Thyatira, your heart has been faithful*
- *Sardis, you have produced only Truth*
- *Philadelphia, you understand and emanate the Truth to others*
- *Laodicea, your vision (energy) is now clear*

This is how you ascend in Frequencies to perfect vibrations! This is astonishing! May we all take this road to heaven's gates.

Once the ceremony is over, end with a prayer of blessings for the group, and set the date for the next one. REEDOO can be used as the traditional Wednesday night prayer meetings or set to commence after church on a Sunday. They could all have lunch together and then begin the session afterward in a more unified spirit. How ever you decide to practice it, please do it unto God.

I hope this book has blessed you. I would love to hear how REEDOO is changing your life and the lives of those around you. Please practice it in sincerity and know that we are commanded to even pray for our enemies. Keep the faith…..and God Bless.

Note: The patterns on the following pages are not the correct size due to the size of the book. Please go to my website at www.breadandwineministries.org and follow the REEDOO link to the free downloads or you can scan and enlarge these to the correct size. Each one was to fit onto a letter size paper.

Blessings…..

Sharon

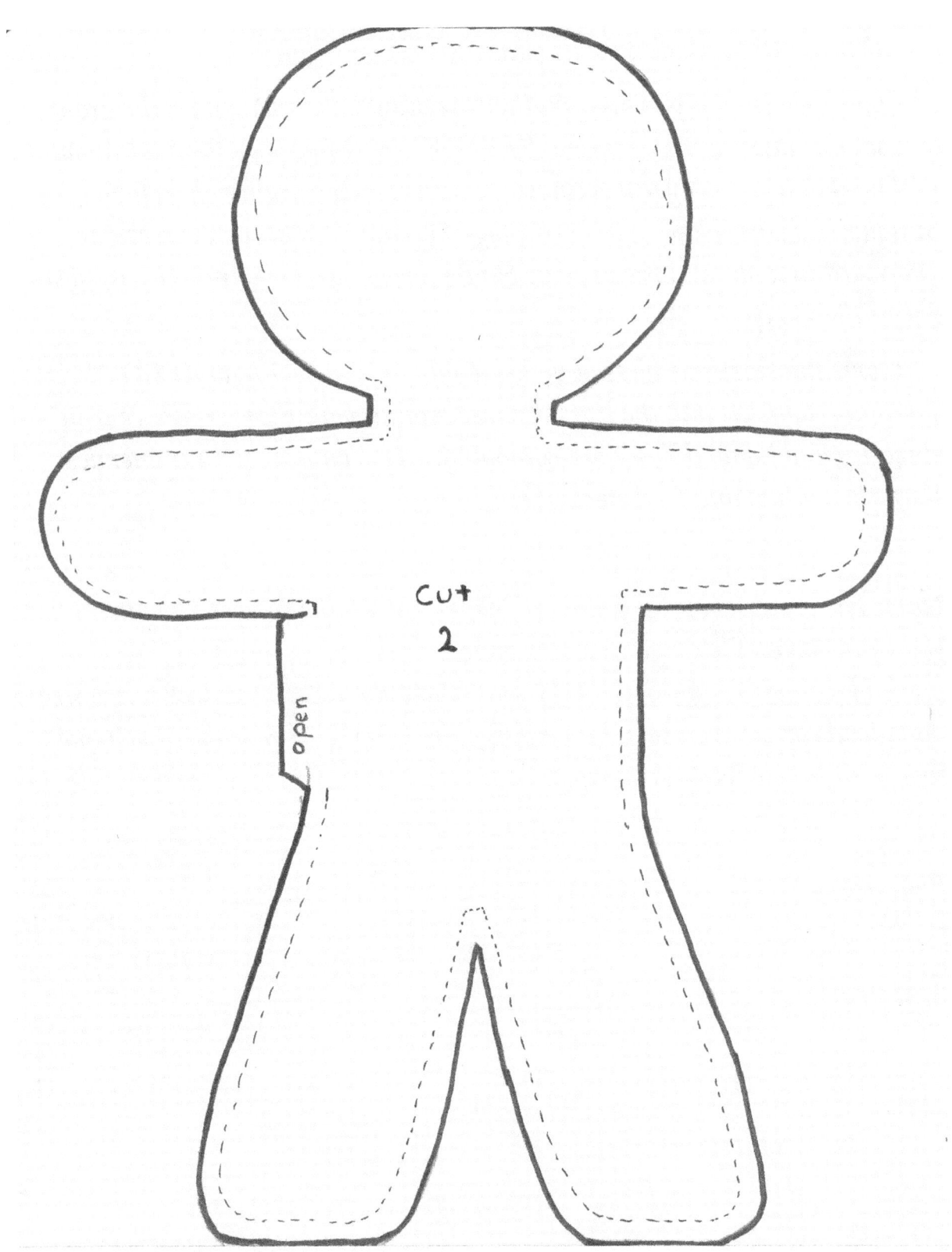

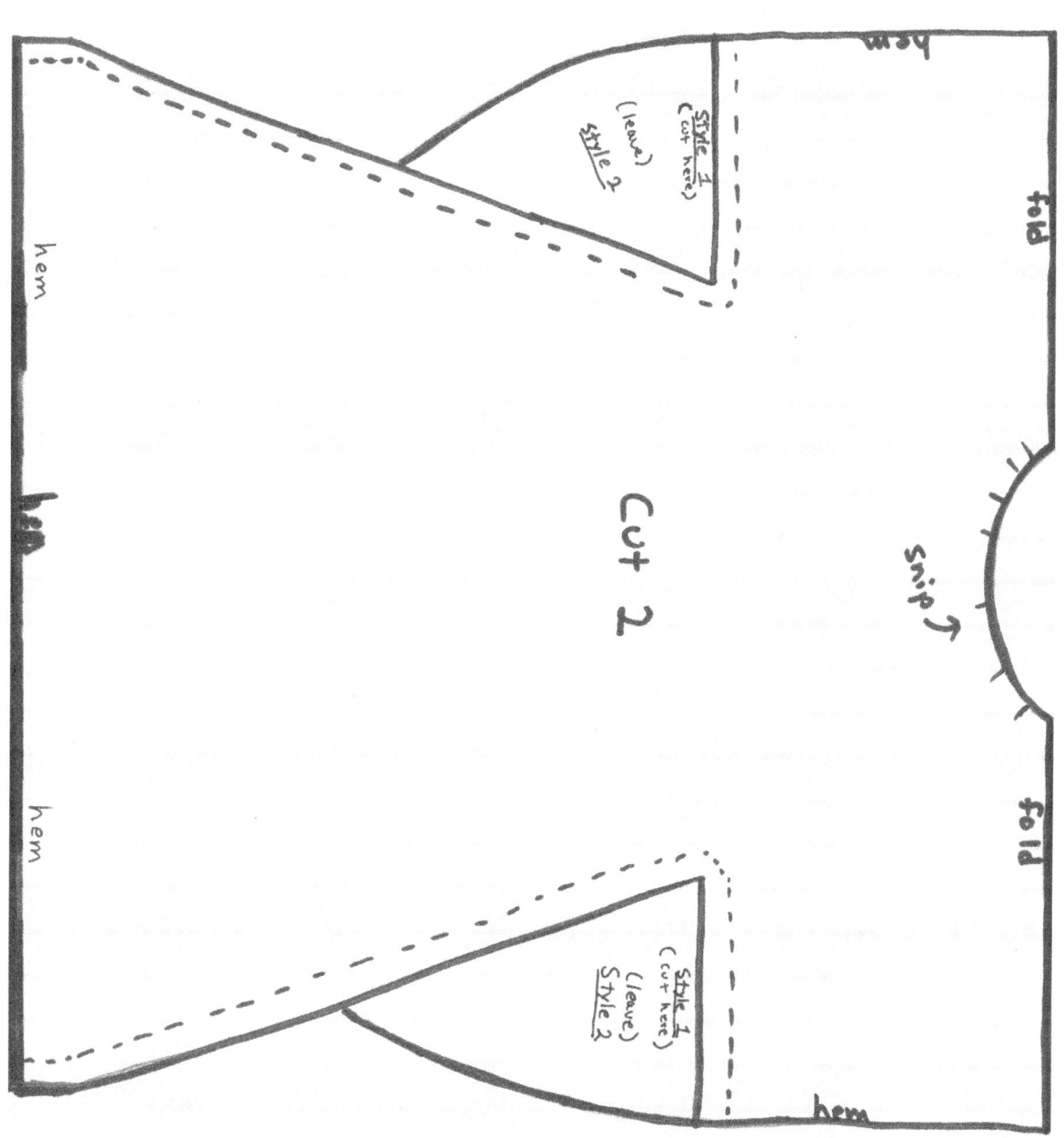

My Journal

www.ingramcontent.com/pod-product-compliance
Lightning Source LLC
Chambersburg PA
CBHW081015040426
42444CB00014B/3217